After the Stroke

Books by May Sarton

As We Are Now
Crucial Conversations
A Reckoning
Anger
The Magnificent Spinster

NONFICTION

I Knew a Phoenix
Plant Dreaming Deep
Journal of a Solitude
A World of Light
The House by the Sea
Recovering: A Journal
At Seventy: A Journal
Writings on Writing
May Sarton—A Self-Portrait

FOR CHILDREN

Punch's Secret
A Walk Through the Woods

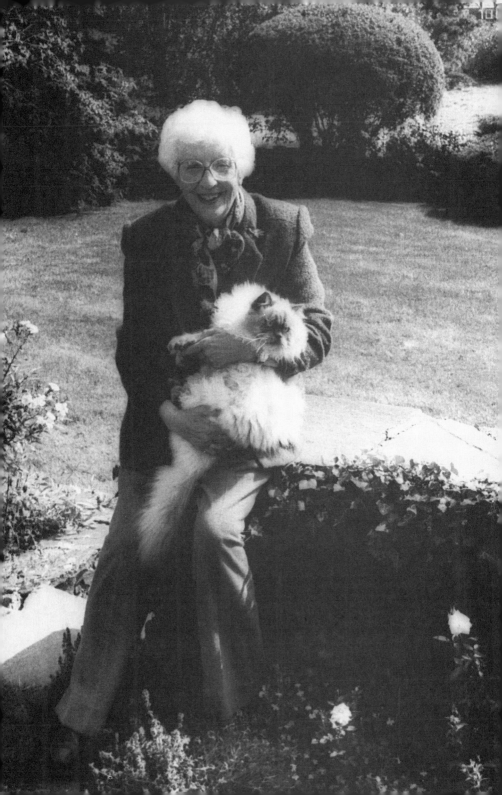

After the Stroke
A Journal

By *May Sarton*

W·W· NORTON & COMPANY · *New York* · *London*

Frontispiece CREDIT: STATHIS ORPHANOS

Endpiece CREDIT: PAT KEEN

The text of this book is composed in Caledonia,
with display type set in Garamont Italic.
Composition by PennSet Inc.
Manufacturing by the Haddon Craftsmen, Inc.

First Edition

Library of Congress Cataloging-in-Publication Data

Sarton, May, 1912–
    After the stroke.

    1. Sarton, May, 1912–   —Diaries. 2. Authors,
American—20th century—Diaries. 3. Cerebrovascular
disease—Patients—United States—Diaries. I. Title.
PS3537.A832Z462 1988   818'.5203 [B]   87–18562

ISBN 0-393-02533-0

W. W. Norton & Company, Inc., 500 Fifth Avenue, New York, N.Y. 10110
W. W. Norton & Company Ltd., 37 Great Russell Street, London WC1B 3NU

1 2 3 4 5 6 7 8 9 0

I wish to thank Vincent Hepp, Nan Parsons, Patience Ross, and Amelie Starkey for permission to quote from personal letters. Grateful acknowledgment is made to the following: Wesleyan University Press, for permission to reprint Part I of "Swimmer" from *The Orb Weaver* by Robert Francis, copyright © 1953 by Robert Francis; The University of Massachusetts Press, for permission to reprint "Invitation" from *Robert Francis; Collected Poems, 1936–1976* (Amherst: University of Massachusetts Press, 1976), copyright © 1936, 1964 by Robert Francis; the *New York Times*, for permission to reprint material from *Critic's Notebook: Right and Wrong Kinds of Love in Theater* by Frank Rich, 10/30/86. Copyright © 1986 by The New York Times Company; Vanguard Press, Inc., for permission to reprint "Lord" from *Long Island Light: Poems and a Memoir* by William Heyen, copyright © 1979 by William Heyen, subsequently issued as a Christmas greeting by William B. Ewert, Publisher, calligraphy by R. P. Hale; the Louisiana State University, for permission to reprint excerpt from *The Flying Change* by Henry Taylor, copyright 1985 by Henry Taylor; Century Hutchinson Ltd., for permission to reprint "An Old Woman Speaks of the Moon" from *Ruth Pitter Poems 1926–66*, Cresset Press, an imprint of Century Hutchinson Ltd; Alfred A. Knopf, Inc., for permission to reprint some lines of poetry by William Allingham from *Come Hither*, edited by Walter de la Mare, 1960; Macmillan Publishing Company, for permission to reprint "Tanist" from *Collected Poems of James Stephen* (New York: Macmillan, 1954).

For Edythe Haddaway
Nancy Hartley
Janice Oberacker

who saw me through

Foreword

UNTIL NOW I have made it a point of honor to add nothing to the daily notations in my journals, and have only revised occasionally for style or to eliminate repetitions. But I was so ill during the writing of the first half of this journal that it became mandatory to enrich it here and there. Bracketed material was written after the given date.

After the Stroke

Wednesday, April 9, 1986

IT MAY PROVE impossible because my head feels so queer and the smallest effort, mental or physical, exhausts, but I feel so deprived of my *self* being unable to write, cut off since early January from all that I mean about my life, that I think I must try to write a few lines every day.

It is a way of being self-supporting. I long for advice from someone like Larry LeShan who is himself recovering from a severe heart attack with many days in intensive care, yet has had the kindness to phone three times, the blessed man. He says I have no surface energy because reserve energy has to be built back first and that makes sense.

Meanwhile I lie around most of the afternoon, am in bed by eight, and there in my bed alone the past rises like a tide, over and over, to swamp me with memories I cannot handle. I am as fragile and naked as a newborn babe.

[I am too vulnerable to all the losses and often the pain connected with personal relationships. I have had too many lives, have attached myself to so many people over the fifty years since I was twenty-five and began my real life after my theater company failed in 1934. It is hard to imagine being able to say "fifty years ago," but during those fifty years I have lived hard and to the limits of my capacity as a human being and as a writer. So it is a huge bundle of feelings and thoughts that ride on those tides when I lie awake at night. My mother dies again, and again I have to face that I did not have the courage to sit with her, which is what she needed. Perhaps

I wrote *A Reckoning* partly to help readers do what I could not do . . . and people write me that it did help.

Then I come back often to Santa Fe where I met Judy on my second visit there when we were paying guests in the same house . . . what a piece of luck that proved to be! Our joining together, our living together in Cambridge was the good end of a long struggle and doubt on her part as to whether she wanted to accept me as a lover and friend. Judy had kept her personal life entirely apart from her professional life as a distinguished professor of English at Simmons College; she hesitated to be pinned down perhaps in the minds of her associates. She was not entirely prepared for the intensity of feeling on her side as well as mine. She was then forty-five and had had no intimate relationship before. And she had suffered from serious depression which she shared with no one until I came along, and even then in all the years we lived together I did not always know when she was in the valley of the shadow. Judy was as inverted and secretive as I am open and indiscreet. What drew us together was mysterious, as true love always is.

Basil de Selincourt was often in my thoughts, the first major critic to recognize my poems, and later a true friend. He looked like a hawk and could be quite brutal. But he read my poems with complete attention all through the years, and wrote his queries to me, and those letters with mine to him are now at the Berg collection with so much else, my correspondence with S. S. Koteliansky for one. It has made me aware that it is men not women who have held my work in high regard, with the one great exception of Carol Heilbrun who came into my life after I was forty-five.

What I see when I think of Basil is his garden in Kingham where he planted hundreds of shirley poppies in a long raised bed, and so made it imperative that I sow some in every garden I have had. I think of his slow walk, the gardener's walk, never hurrying.

And now I go back to find his review in the *Observer* (London) of April 2, 1939, for it was prescient and at the same time and even till now the best present I have ever been given as a poet. Here are two excerpts:

> If her verses deserve notice, it is because the intense experience which underlies and unifies them has engendered an uncompromising determination to forge and refine the tool for its expression, a tool which needed to be, and indeed already is, deep-searching to the point of ruthlessness, and very delicate.

And further on:

> Anyhow, in work like Miss Sarton's—she invokes for it herself the analogy of the spire—"the living spine, the soaring tension"—one claims to know the why of everything, since the more familiar it grows, the more aware one is of its unity of purpose, the more one feels in every line the solemn dedication in which all originated: a kind of dedication peculiarly germane to the poetic outlook in our time. For it grounds the ultimate, creative personality on an ultimate renunciation, on an achieved independence, an impassioned solitariness. Nationalism in poetry is dead. A poet's mind must comprehend all thoughts that visit it, and thoughts pass everywhere today. The poet's voice today becomes the voice of universal reason, and himself a citizen of the world. To be the world's he must first stand alone, must be dead to the world, a spiritual centre, radiating love.

Having been given that at twenty-seven had to sustain me through years of damaging reviews. And of course it did.

But the disturbing, the unresolved memories that flood

me have to do, of course, with love affairs. The fascinating
but sometimes deadly Muses who seem to have brought me
poetry and rage and grief in almost equal measure. Is it perhaps that I have been a bad lover, but a good friend? Or
simply that passionate love at its most romantic and demanding has already the seeds of death in it, the fresh leaves will
inevitably fall in time? At best it changes and grows into
friendship as I am experiencing now in a kind of epiphany
with Juliette Huxley through letters.

When I get overwhelmed by the past I try to force memory
back to rest in landscapes, in places such as the Dordogne
river in France which Judy and I and two English friends
explored just after World War II before it had become fash-
ionable. We were able to see Lascaux, the prehistoric paintings so fresh they looked as though Picasso might have painted
them the day before. Now the government has had to close
those caves to preserve them, and tourists see an imitation,
a reproduction. The region of the Dordogne resembles the
landscapes behind Renaissance paintings. It is rich and gentle
and around every turn of the river brings into view another
small magical castle as in a fairy tale.

All of this and so much more—as they say on television—
is contained in one person, dreaming it all like a dream and
pursued by it sometimes like an inescapable nightmare. No
life as rich can ever be perfectly resolved . . . it can be done
only in a poem or two, only through a work of art. It is too
complex, too terrible, too astonishing and so the wave of memory dashes itself against rocks.]

I have been rather smug perhaps about solitude versus
loneliness—"loneliness is the poverty of self, solitude the rich-
ness of self." Now I am frightfully lonely because I am *not*
my self. I can't see a friend for over a half hour without feeling
as though my mind were draining away like air rushing from
a balloon. So having someone here would not work.

Nancy is a great help. She comes now every day, keeps the bird feeders filled, and works away next door, a beneficent presence, who makes no demands.

Ever since the stroke I often repeat a short poem of Robert Louis Stevenson's which Agnes Hocking taught us at Shady Hill. I learned it when I was eight or nine and did not really understand it. Now I say it at least once a day, and it helps, though it is *not* a great poem at all:

> If I have faltered more or less
> In my great task of happiness:
> If I have moved among my race
> And shown no glorious morning face;
> If beams from happy human eyes
> Have moved me not; if morning skies,
> Books, and my food, and summer rain
> Knocked on my sullen heart in vain,—
> Lord, Thy most pointed pleasure take,
> And stab my spirit broad awake . . .

Thursday, April 10

IF I HAVE learned something in these months of not being well it may be to live moment by moment—listening to the tree frogs all night for I couldn't sleep, waking late to the insistent coos of the wood pigeons—and at this moment the hush-hushing of the ocean. Being alive as far as I am able to the *instant*.

But I think it is necessary before coming back to the present to adumbrate briefly where I am coming *from*.

First an autumn of poetry readings from September through early December—I was riding a wave. And even if it was a bit too much for me, I have no regrets. Would I have missed the great audience at the Smithsonian in Washington, D.C., (sold out months in advance) or across the continent the theater full in San Francisco? Or seeing Moscow, Idaho, in November, when the land lay below a small plane in huge fertile folds, rich black earth—like the body of a mythical goddess—so feminine and restorative an earth, I had tears in my eyes? Would I have missed all that?

[But between readings while I was at home in November, Bramble tried to eat but I realized after a few days that she must have a bad tooth, perhaps an abscess; Nancy and I took her to Dr. Beekman, our vet here in York, an extremely adept and humane man especially where a cat is concerned. I was able to bring her home after a few days, but Dr. Beekman warned me that he had had to take some bone as well as a tooth and the biopsy still to come might, he feared, show cancer of the bone. Her left eye was almost closed.

Bramble always came in at night by climbing the wisteria vine to my bedroom window, often very late at night when I would see her shadow sitting there patiently, waiting for me to open the door to the porch roof, as I could not take the window screen down. She then ran along and jumped across to the porch roof and in. In spring and fall when the screen was off, she jumped straight from the sill to my bed in a lovely leap.

I thought a little later, knowing she could never get well, that the time had come to have her put to sleep, but Dr. Beekman examined her carefully and said, "Let her have another week or so." And so for a last week or two it was a long farewell as she lay full length along my back and purred often half the night. Bramble was always close to the wilderness,

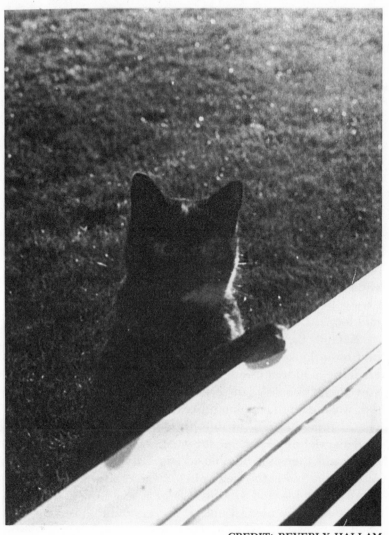

CREDIT: BEVERLY HALLAM

"a long farewell"

the last of the "wild cats" of Nelson, elusive, aloof, but in the end extremely loving.

But when her eye began to look infected again and was closed tightly I decided that we must put her out of her pain and Dr. Beekman assured me that I was right this time. She was lying on her side, perfectly passive, but the right eye so huge with fear, black to its gold rim, so deep and clear, I felt I had never seen such terrible beauty. Dr. Beekman treated her with tenderness, stroked her, called her by name, and then managed to get the needle in with such expertise that she never moved, and in a few seconds she was gone.

Nancy and I were crying so hard we had to wait a moment before driving away and coming home to the desolation here. I often heard Nancy talking her special language to Bramble when she walked Tamas, for Bramble went along, dashing up a tree, bounding through the long grasses like a black and gold leopard. Nancy had loved her too.

Not only the house, but the whole landscape seemed empty, for I often looked out from my study window to see way off down the field that intent black presence waiting for a mouse. Now there was no sign of life. But the worst was going to bed, waking often, thinking she would be at the window, then when I remembered, unable to sleep.]

The grief never left me for weeks. Suddenly I would start to cry and then not be able to stop. What ran through my head was, "this is the beginning of the end." We had been, Tamas, Bramble and I, a little family, and now it had been decimated. Who next? Tamas is so very lame these days and I had been feeling exhausted and ill.

On December twenty-eighth the Christmas tree caught fire—in one second a towering blazing holocaust, black smoke so thick it stifled me as I grabbed a fire extinguisher, calling out to my guest, Judy Burrowes, "Call the fire department! I must stay here and put it out." And that I did, running upstairs to get the second extinguisher when the flames flared up again. Finally when the fire was out the volunteer fire department roared up with an ambulance all ready to take me to the hospital! They were astonished.

The miracle was that the books which are in recessed bookcases in the library, all my own books bound in leather among them, were not damaged except by smoke—but of course it made a frightful mess and took weeks of work to set right—workmen washing the walls, wiping down everywhere: the painters repainting, a new wall-to-wall carpet put down. I couldn't get the saffron yellow of the old one; the new one is rather tame by comparison! Luckily insurance covered most of the damage, including twenty-three hundred dollars to bring the *bahut* back to life.

On December thirtieth I saw my doctor, hoping to get help on the constant intestinal cramps I had suffered on the tour. Instead he discovered congestive heart failure, a fibrillating heart, and put me on drugs to try to get the heartbeat back to normal. The drugs made me really ill—impossible to work—and I had to cancel a spring tour altogether. The cramps became so painful I lay down most of the day, but Dr. Chayka paid no attention to that when I complained.

Then on February twentieth I woke in the middle of the night terrified as I felt as though a numb, perhaps dead, arm were strangling me. It was actually my own left arm. I could not extricate myself. Finally I did manage to and got up— with great difficulty, and staggered about. I knew something was wrong, but went back to bed. At six I called Nancy and asked her to come, went down to let Tamas out as usual, forced myself to make breakfast, carried the tray up to bed, but couldn't eat it. Then I called Janice, my dear friend who is an R.N., and said, "I think I have had a small stroke." She was very firm. "Call your doctor. Get the ambulance—I'll be right over."

It was a great relief when I knew help was on the way. I even managed to pack a small suitcase to be ready, but I could not dress. My left side felt very queer and dead.

Nancy and Janice were both here by the time the ambulance and its two sleepy attendants arrived, and they followed us to the hospital.

What a relief to know I would be taken care of! It had been a hard night's journey into day.

Then followed six days of tests and confabulations. The CAT scan showed a small hemorrhage of the brain—perhaps a clot thrown out by the irregular heartbeat. Then I came home, lucky indeed to be able to speak and take care of myself—the telephone my lifeline. Janice came for one week to get supper and stay the night. Maggie Vaughan came for one week and got all the meals—and then I was alone here again.

It was a *mild* stroke, thank heavens. But what neither I nor my supportive friends could quite realize is how strange one feels—and how depressed—after even a slight stroke— that is what I have been learning slowly for seven weeks.

The absence of psychic energy is staggering. I realize how much it takes to write one line. And I have tried in vain, over and over, to write a poem for Bramble and wept with frustration because poetry is not in me. Will it ever come back? Shall I ever feel whole again?

[Two weeks ago something extraordinary and wonderful happened. I must have mentioned to Carol Heilbrun that if I ever could choose a cat—all of mine have been strays—it would be a Himalayan. She had inquired around and found a four-month-old male kitten and had brought him to me, all the way from New York City. Of course when he finally got here far from his mother and brothers, having been penned up for hours, his one idea was to get away as fast as possible

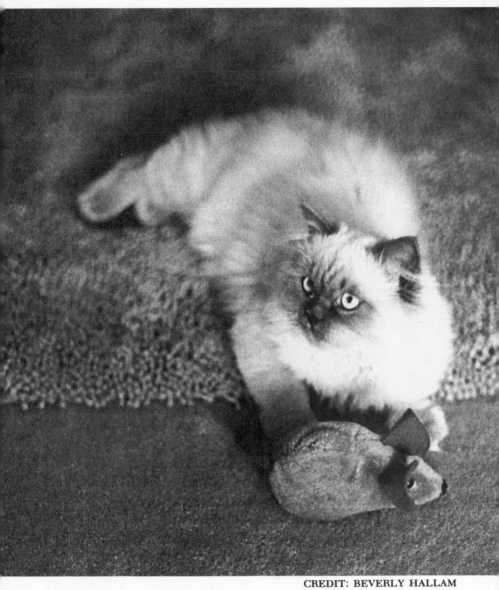

CREDIT: BEVERLY HALLAM

"Mon ami, Pierrot"

and hide. But before he did so I had picked him up and nuzzled the soft fur on his tummy, and had seen his snub nose, his huge blue eyes and his coloring, slate blue face, ears and paws and the rest a creamy white. His paws are huge and very soft. Well, he was indeed a great beauty, but when I went to bed he was nowhere to be found and I wondered and waited and must have finally fallen asleep, for when I woke up before light, I found he was lying on my head and had been there no doubt for most of the night. That was a good sign.

A kitten? At first a hurricane would have been the word. For the first two weeks I was woken at dawn by the sound of a large life-sized stuffed lamb in my bedroom being knocked over, and strange raucous miaows from deep in the kitten's throat as he attacked the beast with claw and tooth, tearing at its tail and ears, then suddenly flinging himself downstairs and racing around the house.

Before he came I had decided to name him Pierrot, "mon ami Pierrot," as he is called in the old song my mother sang to me when I was a baby:

> Au clair de la lune,
> Mon ami Pierrot,
> Prête-moi ta plume
> Pour écrire un mot.
> Ma chandelle est morte
> Je n'ai plus de feu.
> Ouvre-moi ta porte
> Pour l'amour de Dieu.

He had certainly come into my life at a desolate time, when "my candle was out." But at first he did seem in his violence a little too much for me, especially the day after Carol brought him and she had left. For he simply vanished for seven hours, and I did not dare call Carol to see she was safely home until after dark when he suddenly appeared from nowhere and gave a plaintive mew.

That was the beginning and now after two weeks we are semi-friends, routines have been established, and perhaps he and Carol are responsible for my turning the corner at last, and able to begin a new journal.]

Friday, April 11

IT IS STILL COLD and dreary here, although treasures are humping up under the salt hay on the flower beds and maybe by next week I can release them into sunlight. The more miraculous it was, then, in the cold rain, to find yesterday in the mail a tiny box from Duffy in Connecticut containing four sprigs of arbutus, the waxy perfect pink flowers sending out a whiff of that nonesuch perfume—my nose could hardly believe it!

There was also a cassette from a composer, Emma Lou Diemer, at the University of California at Santa Barbara, a recording of her composition for my poem "Invocation"—at its first performance. It was beautiful although the words did not come through, but the musical atmosphere was just right.

At four this morning Pierrot snuggled up under my hand, butting his head into my palm, and lay there purring very loudly—a sweet way to start this day.

He is a ravishing sight, a fluffy white extravaganza and his large, very soft floppy paws suggest that he will become a huge cat.

Saturday, April 12

FROST ON THE grass this morning.

Pierrot decided at four that it was time for a wild tear, up and down and roundabout without stopping for an hour—sliding the scatter rugs under the bed, thumping loudly, scrambling in and out of the bath. At such times his eyes are red; he is a *violent* spirit, a kind of fury and sometimes makes a hoarse, loud, ugly miaow of rage. So by five when it was time to let Tamas out I was tired, but I did get an hour's sleep before I got up at six-thirty and now the sun is out.

It is nine-fifteen. I have done a laundry and cleaned out a big drawer in the kitchen which was full of mouse dirt, a horrid job, and I'm glad to get it off my mind.

When I came home from the hospital after the stroke the daily chores seemed insuperable. Making my bed left me so exhausted that I lay down on it at once for an hour. I realized that I had always hurried through the chores in order to get up here to my desk as fast as possible—it felt strange not to be pressured for the first time since I moved here fourteen years ago—and I tried to learn from it, to learn to take the chores as an exercise, deliberately slowing down, savoring the smoothing of a sheet, the making of order as delightful in itself—not just something to get out of the way.

Often when I lay in bed after my breakfast which I take up on a tray, the light shone through the stained glass phoenix Karen Saum had had made for my seventieth birthday. It always felt like a good augury to watch it glow, blue and red.

Perhaps the phoenix can only begin to rise from its embers when it has reached the very end, death itself. With Bramble's death I felt the wilderness die in me, some secret place where poetry lived. She was so wild—passionate and distant at the same time. When Pierrot comes so easily to be petted early in the morning I remember that it took five years for Bramble to creep up from the end of the bed and lie in the crook of my arm. But then the bond was very deep.

The hardest thing for me to give up after the stroke was writing to Juliette Huxley. Forty years ago we were intimate friends, but time and change intervened, misunderstanding broke the bond, and only now in these last months has she opened the door—and we are communicating again at last. She is eighty-nine. Time is running out—and the frustration of being unable to keep the slight thread intact between us is very hard to bear.

So I made up a dream of flying over to England in June and taking her to a country inn for a few days where we could talk instead of writing. That was the final thing I realized I had to give up. I'm not well enough, and she has had several bouts with flu and herself hesitated to come.

I spent a sleepless night trying to accept that I shall probably never see her again—that was the death of the spirit, the end of dreaming impossible dreams. Strangely enough, the next day I began this journal, and knew that my real self was coming back.

Sunday, April 13

AT LAST a real spring day, brilliant sun, no wind, the ocean murmuring or rather roaring gently in the distance. It made me remember that when I first came here I often thought I heard a train going by—but it was the ocean, not passing through, always to be there.

Having a disability has one good effect. I am far more aware of and sympathetic about the illnesses some of my friends are struggling to surmount than I was when I was well. It is companionable to share some of the day-to-day triumphs and despairs. I'm afraid terribly cheerful, well people are no help at all!

I am aware for the first time perhaps what courage it takes to grow old, how exasperating it is no longer to be able to do what seemed nothing at all even a year ago.

And I am learning some of the things *not* to say to a person who has had a stroke. It's a good idea not to seem to expect great improvement. "Are you feeling better?" when there is no chance that the person addressed *can* feel better quickly. For instance: work. Several people suggested I keep a journal—in the first weeks after February twentieth. This caused me to shout and weep. "I can't write a *line*! I'm not myself and shan't be for a long time." It felt like cruelty—like saying to a cripple in a wheelchair, "it will do you good to take a walk."(!)

A month ago writing a few lines in this book would have been impossible. Will simply had no effect. I had to give up doing anything fast. And the worst has been to have poetry dead inside me—not a line runs through my head.

I have not been able to listen to music at all since early January—perhaps because it has been so closely connected with poetry. I don't dare, for fear of breaking into pieces.

Monday, April 14

WARM SUN and a calm blue sea. Maggie Thomas is here raking leaves along the fence. At eight I got out the rakes, the wheelbarrow, fertilizer and put lime around some of the clematis— but when she got here—such a help!—I was done in as though after a full day of outdoor work. It is so frustrating!

However, Tamas actually walked out and lay down by Maggie in his old place under the maple tree. He has been so lame I was in despair yesterday. So maybe spring weather will give him a lift! And me, too.

Tuesday, April 15

MAGGIE VAUGHAN OVERNIGHT—she comes like Ceres bearing baskets of goodies—applesauce, cookies, thin calves liver, fresh eggs from the farm—cooked our supper although I made an eggplant dish earlier as a vegetable. The thin calves liver

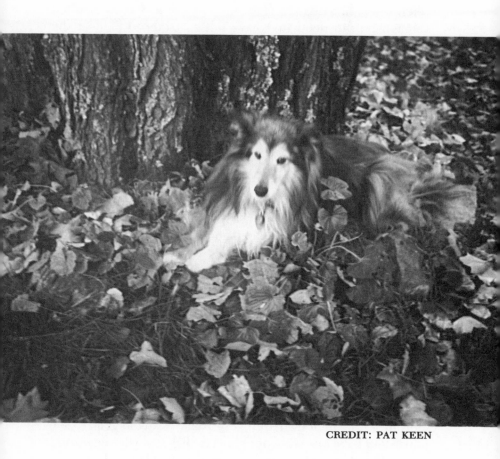

CREDIT: PAT KEEN

was delicious, and for dessert homemade strawberry ice cream, the best I have ever tasted! I feel so cherished and *shielded* when she is here—and before she left she had even brushed Tamas who did need it. I have felt so badly to neglect the dear thing as I have done for lack of energy.

Pierrot played some mild games with her before supper but never showed off one of his wild hurricanes—as he is apt to do early in the morning—instead, slept from five to six nuzzling into my arm.

All this homey peace broken into, of course, by the horrendous news of our bombing of Tripoli and "punishing" Qaddafi by killing at least one hundred civilians and rousing the Arab world against us. What has this outrageous deed of childish reprisal done for us? I feel humiliated, *ashamed.* Now we shall wait for Qaddafi's revenge—then what? Another bombing? More innocent dead? No wonder our allies are dubious. I am unable to say more or even to think. A black day.

Wednesday, April 16

EXPECTING COLD RAIN and wind, we are given another golden morning—but I got overtired yesterday. It was so good to see Janice and have a bowl of her superior fish chowder again and to hear about her exhausting interview yesterday, but we were both too tired really and I was in bed by seven-thirty, then couldn't sleep, too aware at night of what is going on under my skin—fingers of my right hand go numb—my whole head itches, anxiety—another stroke? Absurd, of course.

The good news is that Dr. Chayka has agreed to take me

off Lanoxin—and I hope in a few days to feel *well* after three and one-half months of discomfort all day long. The *drained* feeling in my head is altogether other, the effect of the stroke. But it would be wonderful to enjoy meals, and Scotch—and not feel quite as sick. It has been depleting. I'll see Dr. Petrovich, the heart specialist, on May second—and Janice meanwhile will monitor my pulse—(it may start to race without Lanoxin).

Youth, it occurs to me, has to do with not being aware of one's body, whereas old age is often a matter of consciously *overcoming* some misery or other inside the body. One is acutely aware of it.

I simply never thought about this until the stroke—even when all my teeth had to be removed last year! So I have been lucky. But I see now that the stroke has made me take a leap into old age instead of approaching it gradually.

The kitten is so perfectly at ease inside his body that it is a joy to contemplate him, sometimes lying on his back with back legs stretched straight out and front legs stretched straight over his head. Such ease!

Friday, April 18

YESTERDAY, off Lanoxin and expecting to feel better, I felt so ill I could do nothing but lie around and *wait* for things to change inside my body. So it was especially moving to find a letter about *As We Are Now* in the mail that spoke to me with force.

The writer, Kathleen Daly, S.N.D., wrote in bed with

the flu where she suddenly remembered an experience she had had as a nurse's aide in a nursing home in 1982–1984— and what the novel had meant. She says:

> The relationship you describe between the main character and Mrs. Close had so much likeness to a relationship I experienced that I always find comfort in reading those tender passages. . . . The woman I cared for was eighty-three years old and had had a severe cerebral hemorrhage that left her paralysed on one side and speechless and angry. Her family did not know how to relate to her in this state and were frightened and depressed by her uncontrollable anger and bitterness.
>
> I, having never known her in any other way, fell in love with her. Perhaps I sensed in her anger a spirit that had not yet given up or in her inability to speak (even though her eyes spoke volumes) a voice that needed to be heard and needed help to be heard. (I was experiencing similar things in other ways.) Whatever, I had the gift of caring for her until she died, and at her coffin and at her grave the only words that came to me were 'thank you' and many tears.
>
> She helped me experience myself as tender and compassionate *and* limited. I had to learn how to forgive myself for the many mistakes I made in trying to care for her in the ways that were best for her.

What a wonderful person came into this house yesterday with thanks.

Sunday, April 20

EXACTLY TWO MONTHS since the stroke.

I am at the lowest ebb since December thirtieth when the irregular heartbeat meant the start of taking Lanoxin. It is four months since I have felt well and now I am really in despair—I wake in tears. At this point Pierrot can be exasperating—when he makes a strange guttural mew I know that a fury is taking over—and this morning he overturned a heavy pot with an azalea in it that I was nursing back after the fire—and it took me almost a half hour to clean up the mess.

Later

For anyone who is for any reason feeling weak in the head it is not advisable to suggest solving a problem that requires choices. Yesterday I spent an hour choosing finally a flowering plum tree, from Wayside Gardens, a birthday gift for Mary Tozer and two white azaleas for Anne Woodson. It sounds pleasurable but was actually the hardest hour I have spent for a long time and I cried at the end.

It made me remember going to a friend's from the hospital when I had my tonsils out twenty or more years ago. I felt the same queer sensation in my head as I do now. Then it was from the anaesthetic. This friend gave me a welcome

Scotch and then suggested I plan where to plant a lot of bulbs in her garden. It was an ordeal. Then she gave me ham for supper which I couldn't swallow.

Tuesday, April 22

[ANNE AND BARBARA came over for lunch, bearing egg salad sandwiches as, for once, I could not handle going to get lobsters or making a salad. They came because I felt I must bury Bramble's ashes at last, and we must find a better place for the small soapstone monument Barbara had made for her. We had placed it against the outer terrace wall, but it was covered by snow all winter and I knew we must find a safer, more intimate place, where the plinth with her name and dates engraved on it would not be covered over.

The day was so warm and pleasant that Anne and Barbara sat outside on the terrace steps and ate their sandwiches there. I stayed inside, completely exhausted after we had found the perfect place for the burial, a small recessed plot Raymond had made for me in a crevice between rocks. Gentians have done well there sometimes, but my tries to grow miniature cyclamen failed completely. Bramble will be the presence there now.

After lunch when Anne and Barbara came in to get the tiny box of ashes, I knew I could not go out. I panted after taking ten steps. And more than anything else the inability to help bury my beloved cat's ashes seemed the sign that I was very ill. Later Anne and Barbara told me they thought I was dying. While they worked, and it was a considerable job,

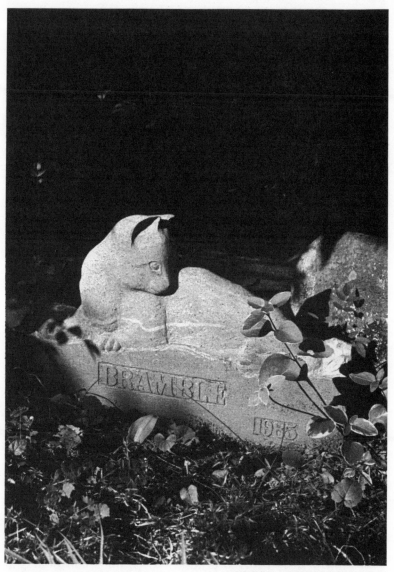

I lay down upstairs, not resting, just bearing the painful cramps.

Meanwhile, Anne and Barbara managed to clear the salt hay off the terrace border and so let some hopeful green shoots breathe.]

Saturday, April 26

A VERY HARD WEEK, I felt awfully sick and lived on ginger ale in sips, and eggnogs. [The cramps had become so debilitating that about all I could manage was to wash the breakfast dishes, make the bed and get dressed. Then I simply lay down for the rest of the morning. Finally I decided that I must make a written plea to Dr. Chayka that something be done about the pain. He did not answer and since this had been going on for months I decided that the time had come to find another doctor. I wish I had done so ages ago, for Dr. Gilroy, whom Mary-Leigh Smart had recommended, listened very carefully to the sad tale, arranged for a barium enema the next day, and called me last night to say that what I have is diverticulitis and he expected it to be cured in a week with Metamucil!

I realized with immense relief that because there had been no diagnosis for four months of great discomfort, I had imagined that I must be dying. This disability had been much harder to handle than the aftermath of the stroke. My left arm and leg are rather weak but it is nothing I cannot manage.

While I rested this afternoon I slept for a half hour and woke with lines of a poem for Bramble running through my head, with ideas pouring out, with a sense of being *myself* again that had left me since January when all this hell began.]

Today I am exhausted, but a reaction was inevitable, I suppose.

Brad Daziel came at nine with a shovel and three rose-bushes for my birthday which he planted there and then. So the rose garden is suddenly rich in promise—it had looked so sad. A gentle damp day, perfect for planting. The daffodils along the woods are out, pushing up through dead leaves. Will it? Can it happen again, I always wonder?

Yesterday at half past three I was still pretty shaky. Bill Ewert came with the poem "Blizzard" he had printed in a special edition and I signed fifty for him. The generous man left many for me and a set of larger ones on water-color paper I can use for gifts. It's a lovely present—and the snow poem becomes a charming spring poem due to his imagination.

Until he came I had felt too tired even to pick daffodils but then on the wave of his friendship I did go out and smelled the delicious damp earthy air.

On Monday Jamie Hawkins came for a brief visit, only the second time she has been here but we correspond. She is a young person for whom I have the greatest respect.

Sunday, April 27

I AM OUT OF BREATH after the slightest effort—couldn't sleep after one in the morning and put a fat pillow behind me—it did help. After I made my bed and did the chores downstairs I was *spent* and lay down on my bed and cried.

Saturday, May 3

MY SEVENTY-FOURTH BIRTHDAY and the fifth month of being ill. Cold today—the daffodils out in the field. Every year I wonder whether they will not have been smothered by the heavy grass, but here they are—bright garlands shining in the still gray-colored field—a miracle.

I am sick and tired of feeling so ill, and of complaining, sick of this old body. Will the electric shock Dr. Petrovich plans set the heart to rights? One more month to wait.

[A strange birthday, the first since I have lived here when it was not possible to have Anne and Barbara for our traditional lobsters. Only Janice came to cheer me up as it began to rain. As always flowers had been delivered but arranging them was an ordeal rather than a pleasure. Has that ever happened before? It made me feel mean-spirited when so many people wanted to celebrate this birthday and give me joy. But I was not there, only a stupid sick animal received them.]

York Hospital, Saturday, May 10

ON WAKING AT SIX I couldn't breathe and, finally after coming home from a liver exam at the hospital and trying to rest, I felt I was suffocating. I called Dr. Gilroy and he put me in the hospital. Heaven to be here, taken care of, after a long wait from five to nine before he came to see me. But *then* I had oxygen and sleep at last. Janice brought me here, and Edythe, always quick to respond in time of need, moved in to take care of Tamas and Pierrot.

I miss Pierrot! Find myself dreaming of his soft paws and the way he stretches out on his back—such a vulnerable position for a little cat! Edythe is enjoying him and, now the sun is out after two weeks of cold, fog and rain, she must be loving to walk out with Tamas among the daffodils.

It is strange that I, on the other hand, have no wish to be there now—only relieved to be here, where I can rest with no chores looming, nothing for which I must summon energy.

Dr. Gilroy took about a pint of fluid out of one lung day before yesterday so I can breathe again.

Now there are weeks ahead of thinning the blood to prepare for the electric shock Dr. Petrovich intends to try when it is safe. If the blood were not thinned another stroke might be in the cards.

Pat Keen will arrive from England for a week on May twenty-second. Somehow we'll manage. I know she will love being here and she knows I've become a Venetian glass aunt— if you remember *The Venetian Glass Nephew.**

From my window I look beyond the parking lot to a beautiful line of trees against open sky. Two are just swelling into leaf, horizontal branches in wide curves. They are my food, my peace, these days. How could we live without trees?

* A novel by Elinor Wylie.

York Hospital, Monday, May 12

HOW I HAVE ENJOYED complete passivity! Being "looked after" like a Paddington bear—listening to the bustle in the corridor as though from very far away so even the noisy voices didn't trouble my floating. But I still feel frightfully tired and so I dread going home.

Meanwhile everyone is ill. Janice had a wisdom tooth extracted and has had awful pain as it got infected. Lee Blair has a small operation on her knee today in New York (just overnight). What next? How fragile we all are—even Janice and Lee who are twenty years younger than I.

And I felt so safe and well. Now I've been knocked down—and that is what is difficult—to be *suddenly* old—to foresee cancelling all public appearances. A radical change of life.

York Hospital, Tuesday, May 13

EDYTHE BROUGHT ME the first copy of Juliette's autobiography *Leaves of the Tulip Tree* with the mail. Such a wonderful thing to happen while I'm still here, undistracted (at home a big order of plants has arrived from Wayside Gardens!), in a safe cocoon of quiet and time. I meant to read slowly but was borne on its tide irresistibly.

It is a very brave, deep and honest autobiography—generous to Julian in more than full measure, but what emerges of course is the rare kind of perception, never sentimental, clear-eyed and highly original in its way of *seeing*, of the extraordinary woman who wrote it. It is time Juliette was recognized as remarkable in her own right.

A lovely bright day here today and I suddenly long to be home and I soon shall be.

Sunday, May 18

THE DAYS ARE CROWDED—too much piles in that I must try to answer, but yesterday I did the *first* real gardening since the stroke—and put in orange impatiens in the shady curve of the stone wall by the Phoenix, some blue phlox, so blue I had taken it for divaricata, in the terrace border, a geum on the yellow side where the wonderful tree peony is very sad. Winterkill everywhere. And now prolonged drought does not help. But everything I want to do takes energy I do not have, so looking at the garden and its needs is a kind of torture.

Still I did sit out on a chair on the terrace after my hour of planting and felt the peace—the birds' evening songs and their swift horizontal flights over my head to the feeder.

I called Vincent Hepp in Houston to thank him for a life-giving letter I got day before yesterday. He has lifted me like a brother over hard places before. He had a much more severe stroke than mine three years ago and this is what he said:

This brings back strange memories to me. A strange trip that I took three years ago, where your fond thoughts and letters accompanied me, a trip from which I returned.

Simple things become impossible. Getting hopelessly tangled putting on my shirt. Desperately seeking the paste for my toothbrush. Turning the wrong button on the cooking range. Burning an empty pan, as my hot water remained inexplicably cold.

People talking about me as they would a child. My power gone, vanished.

Yet this is a trip to the border of wonder world—where words lose their currency, and symbols speak by themselves, as Music would. Time vanishes. I wake up during the dead of night. I sleep at high noon. The most tasteless foods now acquire loveliness: an oatmeal becomes a poem of fragrances. An egg delivers exquisite life to my sick brain.

My most urgent task to do nothing, and find utter satisfaction in it, as my cats, who stretch themselves, lick their dresses, and dream in self-contentedness. And I lie, in the company of the few beautiful things that I really need. A Shakespeare sonnet. An ode by John Keats.

Because I am better off in some ways, I am beaten down by minute "things that have to be done." It is now nine. Pierrot came at a little after five and threw himself down beside me to be cuddled, purred loudly, patted my face, licked it, and we had about twenty minutes of this loving time, a charming way to begin the day. Then I got up, took his very dirty pan down and emptied it, cleaned and refilled it, drank my Metamucil and orange juice, let Tamas out, made my breakfast (oatmeal today with brown sugar and cream), had it in bed with Tamas beside me. He sleeps downstairs these days and I want him not to feel shut out. The difficulty has been Pierrot who hides under the bed and lashes out at poor Tamas when he lies down for breakfast-sharing. So I close the doors: perfect peace. Tamas loves oatmeal!

Then I got up, made the bed, washed the dishes, fetched the bird feeder I keep in the garage at night because raccoons steal it, and hung it up again. Watered the azaleas—everything is terribly dry.

And finally came up here a little overtired already. What oceans of energy I need to have! It astonishes me now even to imagine what I used to be able to do.

Monday, May 19

JUST LIKE VINCENT I left water on the stove for my tea and, when the phone rang, answered and forgot all about it—a favorite saucepan ruined! Everyone says I sound wonderfully myself—but I can't explain that I am not myself and the slightest effort is very costly—I feel excruciatingly tired all the time. So had to give up putting plants in yesterday.

Janice came and attached the long hose for the terrace so I could water the pansies and Nancy, the angel, who is putting in the border of lobelias, can water too, without dragging heavy watering cans from the garage.

I hear the ocean—tide rising—in long comforting roars down there.

Vincent had the extraordinary experience when he had his stroke of writing reams about his childhood. Where did he find the energy? It is mysterious—he might get up at two and write for hours. I have in these four months lived very intensely in the past—Juliette and her presence in my life again in such a caring way has been partly responsible. But I do not *want* to relive the past—can't bring myself to read my letters to her and to Julian which are now in this house.

I want to live in the instant, the very center of the moment—Nancy's voice talking to Pierrot while she plants the plants, and the distant mellow roar of ocean shutting everything less eternal out.

Yesterday Miggy Bouton called about Mother's letters—and talked a little about Mother—how she was able to talk to children so well, on their level, yet never "talking down." So few people alive remember my mother. It was a precious talk with Miggy and brought back good memories of 5 Avon Street in Cambridge, Massachusetts. The Boutons lived across the street and were my "best friends," especially Miggy.

[What a queer state I am in as I see I have not even mentioned the arrival near my birthday of *Letters to May*,* my mother's letters to me which Connie Hunting has published. I made the selection last summer and wrote a preface, and Connie has done a ravishing edition, the cover one of Mother's designs for a book of poems in 1910, the emerald green she loved on a cream background. So all these last weeks I have been happily packing and sending off copies to friends— the best event here in months.]

* Puckerbrush Press, Orono, Maine.

Wednesday, May 21

AT LAST it may be going to rain. A dry wind from the sea was too much and I made myself water the roses and the terrace border where the lobelia Nancy planted was drying out. How I long for energy! Anyway, I made chicken soup for Pat yesterday—it took an hour. The leeks smelled so strong I buried half the bunch in the compost heap! But the soup tasted good, thank heaven! I dragged in a lot of food, fruit for Pat's room, vegetables.

It's annoying that I have to see Dr. Petrovich on Friday at eleven so can't take Pat out to lunch as I had hoped to do and start her visit with what will be our routine.

Friday, May 23

PAT IS HERE, arrived around six yesterday with Edythe who had kindly met her at Logan, as I really could not have stood up for such a long wait. Pat, glowing under her cap of curly red hair, a vivid presence. I felt carried on her energy and sensitive response to everything, including the stuffed animals. "It's a child's house," she said, her eyes sparkling.

What a pleasure, since I again have anorexia from Amiodoroni, to see her eat every bit of the chicken soup I had made, an English muffin and half of mine, and eat her half canteloupe filled with strawberries to the skin! She is going to help me get well. That is clear already.

[As so many of my friends have done, Pat Keen came into my life because she discovered my books at a time when she was fighting severe depression, and began to write me remarkable letters. In these last years my correspondence with Pat is one of the very few I have taken on, because too much comes into the house and short letters are all I can manage. But here was an English actress who lived in Ipswich, Suffolk, where my Grandmother Elwes lived, an actress who had read everything, played several instruments, and was altogether a person of great reality to me.

In November 1984 I went to Belgium for my father's centennial celebration at the University of Ghent, and decided to spend a week or so in London and see Juliette Huxley and meet Pat Keen. Meanwhile Edythe Haddaway had had major surgery and it occurred to me that we must celebrate her recovery by spending that London week together. So for once she was not house-sitting for me, but met me in London after the Sarton centennial. I had several engagements, including a poetry reading at The Poetry Society, and a talk about my work to a class at Jesus College, Cambridge. And unfortunately I had a frightful cold the whole time. Pat Keen saved the day, appeared with a taxi whenever we needed one, got theater tickets for us, and was in general a bulwark against any attack by weather, illness or whatever came about—so dear and helpful a friend that I named her our shepherd.

So, even though I was in no state to receive a guest, I wanted Pat to come here on her way to the opening in Los Angeles of *Nicholas Nickleby*. I wanted her to see this place and to have her first view of the States not Los Angeles but a corner of New England.]

Today I see Dr. Petrovich. Let us hope he has a date in mind for the electric shock—it could be such a relief.

Another gray day with showers promised—we need rain desperately, and today at least the ocean is visible, very gray at the end of the now very green field.

I have parboiled potatoes and onions for the roast lamb we shall have tonight, an easy dinner, and I have a good bottle of Côtes du Rhône to uncork.

Tamas yesterday got into a fit of barking while I waited— from four to six—expecting Pat and Edythe to arrive. I was chasing grackles from the feeders, waved them off for two hours and still they came back—and Tamas barked! An enervating two hours.

The daffodils are nearly over—and suddenly after the spring orgy the florist has very little. How I miss the tulips! Mice devoured at least a hundred here in the garden.

A wonderful letter from K. Martin. She had been to a service in the Unitarian church in Santa Barbara entirely devoted to quoting Sarton. At the end she said, "I will always love you—especially when you said to me, 'You have been to hell and back and you have not realized that this creates a responsibility'." I have no memory of it but I do think it is true. Bless K. for remembering.

Monday, May 26, Memorial Day

IN SPITE of constant cold gray rainy weather since Pat Keen arrived last Thursday, it is wonderful to have her here—and to realize that I can talk happily for hours because I have been starved for this sort of conversation! It is lovely to have this sensitive human energy around.

Tuesday, May 27

ON SUNDAY it cleared halfway and we were able to make our planned journey to see Anne and Barbara in North Parsonsfield. Janice drove us and she is a wonderfully good driver. Not only is a visit to Anne and Barbara always a deep and fulfilling joy and I wanted Pat to meet them above all, but I also wanted her to see that, as one leaves the coast, Maine is full of rural poverty and dying small towns once supported by a shoe or textile mill—and how much uncultivated land there is everywhere, or woods—owned by whom, one wonders?

We brought lobsters—Pat's first and she did a remarkable job of eating every possible scrap.

Only a few birds at the feeders at lunchtime—I had hoped for the evening grosbeak and maybe one of the eight bluebirds nesting in the bird boxes in the field. But we did see a ruby-throated hummingbird—also Pat's first.

And of course there was wonderful conversation as always, ranging from the peace and the life there to Pat's forthcoming tour of the U.S. with *Nicholas Nickleby*.

Edythe had come to look after the animals and the good day ended with a homey pizza with her. I had had a half-hour rest at Anne and Barbara's before lunch so felt triumphant to have achieved such a long good day and *not* feel exhausted.

But yesterday was bad. I felt really ill in the afternoon after lunch at the York Harbor Inn, looking out over a spar-

kling ocean with almost no one there so we could talk in peace.
But all afternoon I felt very queer again and could not eat a
mouthful of the swordfish we had for supper. Pat, thank goodness, enjoys anything I have to offer. A wonderful guest who
feels like family. I realize how lonely I have been.

Friday, May 30

PAT HAS GONE off for two nights to Edythe Haddaway who
will take her to Newburyport and Salem. So I have forty-eight
hours in which to get household things sorted out—and myself
centered. It has been a wonderful and nourishing visit but
rather an effort.

Yesterday I went into a tailspin. Luckily Pat was not here
to hear me sobbing and howling with rage and despair. On
Friday they did a rhythm exam and it showed a very accel-
erated heartbeat, so Dr. Petrovich has put me on double
Lanoxin and the experimental drug Amiodoroni for three days.
Yesterday was the second day and when I lay down after lunch
I began to have excruciating pain (worse than menstrual pain)
in my lower abdomen. By three I was exhausted, so I went
down to call one of Dr. Petrovich's nurses, a kind woman
called Lucy, to say they must give me a painkiller if this torture
has to be prescribed again. Meanwhile when I sat on the porch
to make the call (I did not have the number by my bed), I
found two swarms of flying ants crawling all over the door and
the window behind me *inside* the house. One kind is an inch
long!

Lucy calmed me down somewhat, and then I went out,

having remembered that Karen was sowing seeds in the annual garden, and screamed for help. Karen reminds me of *Le Grand Meaulnes*—she is so thin and tall. She came running and together we swept the ants into paper bags. I finally used Raid to kill off those that were left. This is the second time this spring I have suffered this horrifying invasion.

It is unbelievably wonderful that Karen was willing to come back from Tucson and work for me this summer. No longer do I see a thousand things that need doing and know I cannot do them—and she is so happy to be here! When I suggest that she had better stop at the end of the day she says, "Oh I'm so happy, I can't bear to leave!" I feel wonderful support from her and from Nancy who helped me change the sheets on my bed this morning. Dear helpers, dear friends.

Life in the country is always a battle against nature, so to speak. For example, this has been the worst year for winterkill since I came here nearly fifteen years ago. The tree peonies, my pride and joy, have almost no buds and are about half the size they were. Red squirrels ate almost all the buds of the big white rhododendron at the back—the day after I had seen how big and fat the buds were and rejoiced. Mice, voles or chipmunks ate fifty tulip bulbs from the terrace border, twenty from the shady border where the begonias are, twenty at least from the narrow upper border on the terrace. Only along the fence about twenty survived. Fifty were eaten in one end of the picking garden. Altogether a disastrous year.

I have reached again a hard place in my illnesses. I am on the edge of anger all the time. Lonely, desperately when no one is here, and then exhausted if anyone is. I seem to be an impossible person who, as Marynia Farnham used to say about certain people, should be shot at dawn.

All the people who have always had instant response from me still expect to—and they are not few. So instead of keeping this journal, I try to answer—and instead of answering well as I used to, break down and cry because I can't.

I have not been able to listen to music since early January but now I have put the Fauré *Requiem* on, and as I listen I see I must listen. I must get celestial food again and try to live on another plane, get down deep enough so all this doesn't matter.

Monday, June 2

LAST NIGHT we went over to Beverly and Mary-Leigh so Pat could see *World of Light*, the beautiful documentary film Martha Wheelock and Marita Simpson made about me some years ago. It was during a thunderstorm which lasted for *five hours*. I went home after the film and left Pat to be introduced to Mary-Leigh's and Beverly's treasure house of paintings and works of art. With the wild storm outside it seemed rather a long visit, so at eleven I called and suggested she had better come home. At times lately I sound and behave like my grandmother who could be rather sharp. Oh dear. Pierrot was a great help, unafraid of the blazing flashes of lightning and roars of thunder, he lay on his back beside me purring loudly.

Wednesday, June 4

DURING ONE of our long good talks I said to Pat, "I must somehow get onto another plane"—and this morning when I woke at five I decided to lie there and think of all the good things in my life now. One is surely waking in my wide bedroom, with its casement windows (which I believe resemble those at Wondelgem where I used to wake as a baby) and sense of space and light. The light I see first is the brilliant blue and red of the stained glass phoenix which hangs high up on the glass door to the outdoor porch. Then if I look to the left my eyes rest on "the hills of home," an abstract painting over the fireplace that Anne Woodson painted using, as though buried under those hills, ancient slate headstones from the Nelson cemetery. Above the hills, a solid blue sky.

The big curtains at the windows are drawn these days as it is light so very early.

On my left is a round turntable with rows of medicines on the top and two layers of books below—and these days a square wicker stool also covered with books. Medawar's autobiography these nights, interesting and lively, but not to be compared with Juliette's as a work of art. There is Mary Barnard's new book of poems written around the astral myths, and Henry Taylor's *The Flying Change* which has just won the Pulitzer prize—how happy I was when I read that he had won it, and he writes me that it came as a *total* surprise!

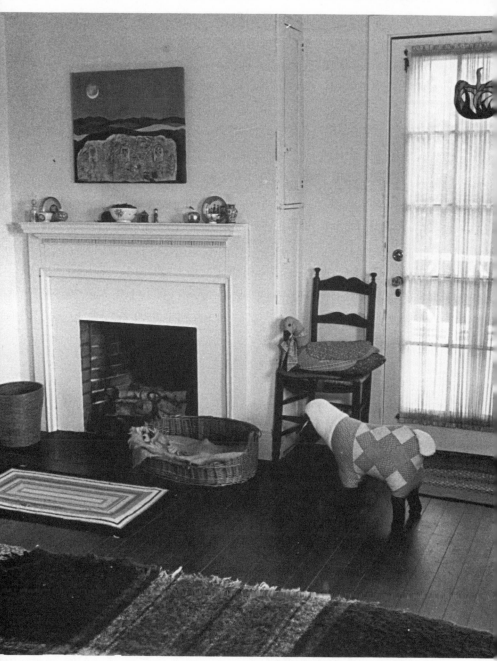

CREDIT: BEVERLY HALLAM

I read it through in one sitting with tears streaming down my cheeks to be with true poetry again—and have just gone back to the last lines of the title poem:

> I see that age will make my hands a sieve;
> But for a moment the shifting world suspends
> its flight and leans toward the sun once more,
> as if to interrupt its mindless plunge
> through works and days that will not come again.
> I hold myself immobile in bright air,
> sustained in time astride the flying change.

Above the round table there are two calendars of the English countryside which I always order and always enjoy and somehow *need*—for England and these landscapes are in my bones.

Pat said she felt at home here partly because I and the house are so European, and I felt at home with her for the same reason.

Thursday, June 5

AFTER THE LOVELY MOMENTS of waking comes the reluctant tug every morning to get up and get going. It is now nearly half past nine and the "getting going" has taken almost three hours—partly because Eleanor Perkins is here cleaning and I have to tidy things up a bit more than usual. I went downstairs at a little after six to let Tamas out, set the tray for my breakfast (cream of wheat this morning), fetch the bird feeder from the garage, refill and hang it up. Then I offered Pierrot breakfast which he didn't want, eager to go out and chase chipmunks.

I then went back to bed and dozed for an hour. Finally got up at seven, made my breakfast and, with Tamas preceding me, carried the tray up to have it in bed. Tamas lies beside me and wants to lick the bowl, and is given small treats, dog snacks, meanwhile. A friend who saw my tray all set and didn't know about this asked, "Do you eat dog biscuits for breakfast?"

That time in bed after drinking my *café au lait* is precious. I sometimes lie there thinking for a half hour. Today I had to get up, before I was ready, to tidy up the guest room (take vases of dead flowers down, etc.) and wash the week's towels in the washer on this floor. That was a bright thing I did for once (I am such a bad housekeeper)—to have it installed so nearby.

Then I still had to wash my breakfast dishes, rearrange flowers—I picked a few Star of Bethlehem, and five English bluebells to make a little magic, and added in some tiny lavender carnations I found at Foster's yesterday. It worked.

Soon there will be peonies to pick in my garden. But the chipmunks have decimated the rhododendruns. It is *very* hard to accept this, as it would have been a glorious year and so much else suffered during this hard winter.

Writing this account of morning chores does make me see that I am better—although, when I finally got up the two steep flights of stairs to my study, I felt that strange drained exhaustion as though energy were a solid substance and had suddenly melted away.

Tomorrow I see Dr. Petrovich and we'll see what he has to say. I can't remember what it was like to feel *well*.

Friday, June 6

A DISMAL DARK DAY, raining hard. Pierrot, who is in a state of ecstasy and frustration chasing the chipmunks he never catches, wanted to go out into the wet wild world, and out he is.

I went to sleep thinking of Sakharov and woke up thinking of him, what being locked away in Gorky and totally vulnerable means—at least once the KGB has come and tortured him. This could happen at any moment. One hears that he is close to being a saint, the most gentle man imaginable.

Amnesty International's twenty-fifth anniversary yesterday. They have a remarkable record partly because they single out individuals and put up an intense barrage over him or her. Millions of others, not chosen, have no hope of course. I find I give to A.I. all I can.

If only Sakharov could be freed!

Animals and birds, except for the shrike, a bird who impales small birds in order to eat them later, as far as I know do not torture each other, and especially do not torture members of their own species. The fact that man does and has done for centuries remains horrifying—and of course we know more and more about what amounts to sexual torture within marriages. Give a person power over another person and the ease with which he uses it to punish is staggering—hardly aware of what he is doing—and if I use the masculine pronoun here it is because in spite of feminism so many women lack

power because in our society money is power. I see it so
clearly in my parents' marriage—the absolute power the money
he earned gave my father when my mother was doing all the
housework and he never realized what food, clothes, etc. cost.
It is hard for me to forgive—

So let me turn away and toward old age, the Fourth Season, as it has been called. How many times lately someone
my age or older has said "if they had told us what it would
be like we would have opted out". Both Polly Starr and Molly
Howe, roughly ten years older than I, have had implants
which have *not* restored the vision so far. Eleanor Blair, now
ninety-two, and legally blind, broke her left wrist and learned
to cook with one hand—her faithful cleaning woman comes
every morning on the way to work to help her do her hair
and dress. Charles Feldstein's wife, Janice, has some dreadful
trouble with her legs and has to be in a wheel chair. Annie
Caldwell, poor dear, has had to suffer a hugely swollen arm
after her mastectomy.

Among all my old friends only Patience Ross, who was
my English agent as well as my friend since the thirties, is
rejoicing. But there is the change over from the long years
with her friend Louise Porter to a happy new companionship.
Patience says, "I only *feel* old physically. Life continues full
of discoveries, some being made *so late*. (But I can't agree
with Oscar Wilde!) I'm hideously lazy and self-indulgent and
enjoy, enjoy—"

I've been going back to Ruth Pitter in my mind and reread a poem I have loved:

An Old Woman Speaks of the Moon

She was urgent to speak of the moon: she offered delight
And wondering praise to be shared by the girl in the shop,
Lauding the goddess who blessed her each sleepless night
Greater and brighter till full: but the girl could not stop.

She turned and looked up in my face, and hastened to cry
How beautiful was the orb, how the constant glow
Comforted in the cold night the old waking eye:
How fortunate she, whose lodging was placed that so

She in the lonely night, in her lonely age,
She from her poor lean bed might behold the undying
Letter of loveliness written on heaven's page,
The sharp silver arrows leap down to where she was lying.

The dying spoke love to the immortal, the foul to the fair,
The withered to the still-flowering, the bound to the free:
The nipped worm to the silver swan that sails through the air:
And I took it as good, and a happy omen to me.*

Saturday, June 7

RAINY, foggy like yesterday—dismal weather for early June
and I feel low, pushed by the need to be up here at my desk.
  The lowest day for a long time.

Monday, June 9

IT GAVE ME A SHOT in the arm to offer a glass of champagne
to three women who had been at the H.D. centennial celebration at Orono this week. It was Diana Collecott who had

* *The Spirit Watches*, Macmillan, 1940.

asked to come and Silvia Dobson and her friend had offered
to drive her here on their way to Philadelphia. After all the
rain and loneliness I felt warmed by their pleasure in being
here. And what a delight to learn that D.C. teaches me at
Durham University in England in a course on American women
poets! She talked a lot about my correspondence with H.D.
I had forgotten how many letters there were—but she wondered why there were comparatively few from H.D. Now
Nancy has helped me find four more in various books of hers.
What would I do without Nancy who knows where everything
is?

Today at last a clear June day—it seems unbelievable, for
it is only the second time this spring that I have picked flowers.
I went down to the annual bed because the yellow day lily
that always flowers first is in flower, and picked some and a
dark purple iris. I seem to have escaped through the long wet
grass without a tick. They are extremely healthy and numerous
this year. To this I was alerted when I discovered a whole
covey in Tamas's poor ears. After that Nancy and I check him
every morning, and I do it at night too. Apparently the cat,
white as he is, does *not* attract. That is a real help as his fur
is so long and thick.

Diana, with whom I had lunch alone, says the poems are
really getting through in England—partly because the paperback *Selected Poems of May Sarton* can be bought (she
assigned it in her course)—and she was excited about pos-
sibly publishing the H.D.-Bryher-Sarton correspondence and
had copied out parts of my letters to Bryher about H.D.'s
poems.

Janice came at four for a good catch-up—I have not seen
her for ages—and to weed her vegetables (she is using half
the annual bed), and brought me the first fruits, two radishes,
when she had finished.

It was a good day but I was pretty tired by the middle of

lunch. I could not eat at all—only a glass of milk and a pretence of eating a clam roll. Pierrot had a little nap with me and that was a great help.

Afternoon

A moment of pure joy, as I lay in the *chaise longue* for a few minutes—it was four. The afternoon light struck two sprigs of mountain laurel, so richly white, in a brilliant blue glass vase—the whole room was filled with their presence and I just lay there and looked. Duffy who sent arbutus in April (what a miracle its pungent scent seemed) had sent the mountain laurel in a box.

Tuesday, June 10

A PURE JUNE DAY. An early pale pink single peony is out and I picked two, and one velvety deep blue Siberian iris this afternoon. But it is a dismal afternoon inside me, so tired I am of never feeling well; I expect the double dose of Amiodoroni is beginning to poison my system. It does not, however, give me the violent cramps Lanoxin did, thank heaven. I am on the fourth day of seven on the double dose.

This afternoon I felt too sick to be able to rest. It has gone on so long, five months and a half, that is why it gets to me—and so little hope. Why do I trust Dr. Petrovich? He has been talking about electric shock for months. Is he just an experimenter with drugs? I do not feel I am being treated as a whole person or that he has the slightest idea what it is for me not to be able to work.

This afternoon I felt almost ready to go to a major hospital—everyone outside thinks I'm crazy as a loon not to.

Wednesday, June 11

EDYTHE BROUGHT delicious veal stew for supper and lemon pie. I could only eat a few mouthfuls but it was a feast day for Tamas and Pierrot, and since Edythe loves the animals she didn't mind.

Yesterday was a fine day but today rain *again*! It is hard because Karen Olch has had to take several days off and now again a whole day is lost. But she has already done wonders in the garden. The strange bronze tree peony has one flower out and the other peonies are on the brink now.

Two remarkable letters, one from Montana, the other from Oklahoma yesterday. From Montana, an artist, who inherited from her father a rough piece of land in an old mining town which had been used as the town dump. How thrilling to read:

> We pitched a tipi amid the rubbish—the cans & broken glass—an old shoe, a purse, a broken toy, the dead car bodies & a horse whose rotting fragrance filled the air on the hot days of that first summer. These bits & pieces, discarded from other's lives became, quite literally the ground, the foundation of our new one.

She goes on to tell what has happened since in twelve years:

> In these twelve years, many people have come & gone and helped to build "the place" as it is now—a large

fenced garden, 2 small cabins & a big house of logs & timbers, the goat shed (now used for storage) and most recent & most exciting—the studio of my dreams. It's large (20 by 40 ft.) and snugly built with high ceilings & a clear-story [sic] for north light.

And it's here I sit to write you, this morning full of bird song & sunlight. (Nan Parsons, Basin, Montana)

She wrote me because of *At Seventy*.

Thursday, June 12

THE RAIN LET UP briefly yesterday afternoon but now it has become a steady downpour. My next to last day on two Amiodoroni a day—the end is in sight.

Never have I been more aware than in these last months how life-preserving my routine is. The day becomes a series of stepping stones—from breakfast to household chores, to coming up here to my study for an hour or so, then the change of pace and relief of driving the car down to the town to get the mail and do errands. I get back very tired, and there is Tamas eagerly awaiting his one dog meal of the day. I'm afraid he has quite a few people meals as he licks my plate at lunch and dinner and these days I can eat almost nothing. Next stepping stone, I lie down on my *chaise longue* and read the mail, which often takes an hour and sometimes—so many people depressed or ill or in need!—is too much for me. But after lunch—often chocolate milk and a peanut butter sandwich on thin bread because I am lazy—I fall on my bed and go to sleep at once. After taking a Coumadin and waking an hour later, I lie there for a while considering what to do—and read the paper with a glass of orange juice and Metamucil—then climb the stairs to this study once more, sort out the mail, see what Nancy can answer for me tomorrow, and maybe write one letter.

At half past five, next stepping stone, put on the local television news and get my supper together. The last stepping stone is doing the dishes and by eight I am in bed—these days reading with the utmost interest the meaty and fascinating long biography of Helen Waddell. I haven't read as absorbing and nourishing a book for ages.

Between twenty and thirty Helen Waddell had to give up everything she wanted—including a fellowship to Oxford, seeing her friends, going to dances, leading a normal young woman's life—to take care of her extremely selfish and ungiving stepmother who took every sacrifice for granted. Ten years of this imprisoning of a free spirit, and a gifted one! Even reading about it is hard to bear. But she managed to graduate from the University of Belfast with high honors, nonetheless. Yet what comes through, too, is her own belief that nothing worth winning is going to be easy. She and her eight brothers and one sister were brought up as children in Tokyo . . .

So the routine makes a frame and I feel that there *is* a next stepping stone to force me to do something, helps me get through the hours when I feel simply ill, passively and hopelessly ill.

The animals are also a help—even looking for ticks on Tamas becomes a kind of game. And Pierrot's wild antics tell me "to hell with your routine—I want to fly downstairs and play!" Fly he does, his feet not touching the steps, or so it looks.

Pat called from Los Angeles to tell me the dress rehearsal,

given for theater and Hollywood people, was a triumph. They stood and cheered at the end of each part—the whole thing takes eight hours! This news cheered me immensely.

Friday, June 13

STILL POURING! "Wildness and wet"—Pierrot is in a frenzy of frustration—and so am I. Due at the dentist in Portsmouth for the cleaning of my two remaining teeth—and also to do errands. It's a rare thing for me to drive so far and stay away so long—and unfortunately I have to stop on the way at the hospital for a blood test ("pro-time" they call it).

Yesterday—rain *all* day. Karen Olch came and spent the day cleaning out the plant window, washing and pruning plants, feeding them, clearing out some of the detritus that accumulates—and even washing the windows! It makes an enormous difference in the whole feel of the room, neglected as it has been for months.

Karen is a treasure—a very careful and thorough workman who shames my casual ways.

Sunday, June 15

THE EFFECT of the last days on two-a-day of the drug has been devastating, and after a hell of a day yesterday I woke even worse off this morning. I'm glad I managed to go out for dinner with Nancy and to the movie *A Room With A View* as planned. I felt awfully sick all through it but it's visually a marvelous work of art and made me very nostalgic for Italy, for Florence where I spent May of my nineteenth year.

Afternoon

Unfortunately I felt Bonham-Carter was miscast as Lucia— L. *must* have character and that pudgy little face lacks just that.

For only the second time this spring I sat out on the terrace at four and drank my orange juice and Metamucil—lots of sails on a hazy blue ocean, and as always at that time lots of birds all flying south, some only to my feeders just south of the terrace. I chased a huge gray squirrel off one of them before I came out. Poor Karen said something is eating the tops of her seeds as they push up, cosmos among them. Snails? I wonder.

On Friday—and it did finally clear up after all the rain— Karen Saum came at four-thirty bearing our supper: swordfish, lettuce and aspargus from the garden where she is house-sitting, a melon and Camembert! What a feast. It was feast enough to see her and we had a good long talk.

But I could hardly eat one mouthful when she served our supper, so it turned out to be a feast for Tamas and Pierrot—and I burst into tears of shame, so awful it felt after all the loving trouble Karen had taken.

Things are not easy at H.O.M.E. but she never wavers in her dedication, and she looked radiant. One of her sons is teaching Spanish there this summer and her mother will come in July. So many of my friends do have family, it feels strange sometimes to have none, as though I am at the center of an immense emptiness—alone.

Will the time come when I can listen to Mozart again? What keeps me from playing records, like a finger across my mouth? The fear of a complete howling crack-up? Or that poetry would then seize me and shake me to pieces like a wild animal with prey? Who knows?

Friday, June 20

I'M ENTERING a new phase. Monday and Tuesday were very hard days. On Monday I simply stayed in bed, feeling too sick to make the effort even of getting up. Nancy, the wise one, persuaded me to call Dr. Petrovich's office and tell one of the nurses, who said at once, "We'll find time tomorrow for you to see the doctor," and it was set for four-thirty. When he saw how upset I was, and close to despair because of *never* feeling well, he suddenly asked, "How would you like to have the cardioversion tomorrow?" It felt like a reprieve and of

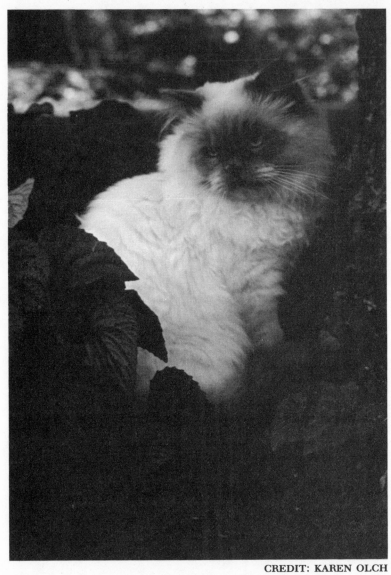

"face like a crumpled pansy"

course I hummed with hope and said, "Yes, by all means."

[Cardioversion is an electric shock which often gets the heart back in sync when it has been fibrillating. Of course I was a little nervous lying on a narrow bed in Intensive Care for a half-hour or so before Dr. Petrovich arrived and the machinery could be set up. Then I was alone again and by now quite tense.

I decided to invent a game of visualizing, a flower perhaps, but finally I decided on Pierrot's face and slowly brought it into focus in my mind, thinking, "It looks like a crumpled pansy," and I smiled because it really does. I felt pleased to have invented a device against nervous tension.

When the cardioversion finally took place I was anaesthetized for a few seconds and it was over.] Dr. Petrovich said, "It's fine. It's done the trick!" Euphoria! I was a prisoner set free. And for an hour I lay there in bliss waiting for a sandwich and a glass of milk—it was near two.

But then when a nurse brought me *the* pill, Amiodoroni, the one that makes me ill, I realized I was being asked to go back to hell. It was a traumatic reversal and a storm of tears popped out of me. Late that night, around nine-thirty, after I had gone to sleep, now in a private room with the same lovely view I had had before of a line of trees against the sky, Dr. Petrovich came in. Yes, I have to take the pill or have another stroke. The hardest thing psychologically to take is that he does *not* believe this drug makes me sick. He insisted it was the fibrillation that did. So I am on the drug, one a day for a week, then one every other day.

Dr. Gilroy also came in to see me and said if I am still as miserable in two or three weeks to go and see him. This was comforting.

I woke to nausea and begged for something to help, and they did give me something which unfortunately made me very groggy all day.

Edythe fetched me at the hospital and it was a help to have her here last night. We had fun making a homey supper together of corned beef hash with a poached egg and a little salad, half a grapefruit for dessert. We watched Pierrot play.

But that night in the hospital when I lay and tried to face what must be accepted, I realized that a kind of aloneness is with me now. I have to curl up deep down inside myself. For the moment I have no energy even for the telephone. This is a new phase as I wrote at the start today—a phase in which I am more alone than ever before.

A steady downpour outside this morning matches my mood and I rather like this wild, wet world.

Monday, June 23

AGAIN SATURDAY and Sunday I gave up and stayed in bed. I see clearly that the psychological problem is that I see *no change*—with an operation one gets better, some hard days, but the movement is there towards healing. If I had terminal cancer I would be on my way elsewhere, movement of another kind. But for five months I have been on a plateau of misery.

So something has to change and I have made an appointment with Dr. Gilroy for tomorrow.

York Hospital, Tuesday, June 24

AS AGREED I stopped in at Dr. Petrovich's office yesterday morning for Lucy to give me more pills—Amiodoroni—and to listen to my heart. She was upset to find it was back fibrillating and called Dr. Petrovich at once—he has put me back in the hospital, has put me on three-a-day of the pill and will do another cardioversion of the heart on Saturday. I was happy to be back in shelter again, not responsible for *anything*—for Sunday evening I had got stupidly exhausted catching Pierrot—it's his evening game to run in and out of the bushes playing hide-and-seek. Before that I had chased a huge gray squirrel off the big feeders eight times, running out with Tamas behind me, barking—and back again out of breath. I shall be missing the peonies at their height, but the truth is I have been too sick to enjoy the garden or to pick flowers. I can hardly believe it.

What I have enjoyed is the wonderful silence at night— the steady throb of tree frogs and crickets and far away the long crescendos of gentle surf as the tide rises and ebbs. So it is not silence but a soothing, comfortably peaceful sound.

But here in the hospital I look out again on the line of trees which were leafless in April and are now rich and dense in their leaves, great green humps against the sky.

I have been pretty depressed because it looked as though there were no avenue open from this plateau of illness I have lived on for months. But when Dr. Petrovich came in yesterday after lunch, he told me that there is still a last resort for which I would have to go to Massachusetts General for an operation that would readjust the heartbeat and make possible a pacemaker. So I have a new hope. Another few weeks, and maybe. . . .

Yesterday I finished Frances Partridge's last journal, *Nothing Left To Lose*. I hated so much to finish it and may read it again. A journal like this becomes a whole life one lives with, and in it I saw very well that what makes a good journal so moving is not the big events but tea in the garden or its equivalent.

York Hospital, Wednesday, June 25

I FEEL DRUGGED and exhausted today, but if it is the effect of the tranquilizer I am now taking three times a day with Amiodoroni, it is at least better than the previous nausea and pain.

Outside I look out happily on the green mounds of the trees moving slowly in the wind—and a sky full of lovely wind clouds. The hospital is heaven, I am so tired. But I have nothing as good as Partridge to read. Helen Waddell is too long, and a newly translated South American novel Joan Palevsky sent a bit too much for me in my present mood.

Thursday, June 26

DIFFICULTY IN BREATHING, so I have oxygen now but the heartbeat is still 110–120—and am very glad to be in the safe cocoon of the hospital *again*.

York Hospital, Sunday, June 29

THE SECOND HEART conversion was done about eight-thirty yesterday morning—again a success, and feeling so *well* all day, able to breathe and think of what life can be like again, if this time the conversion *sticks*. Heartbeat 84 this morning (it reached 130 after I got to the hospital).

Yesterday I finished the biography of Helen Waddell— and am glad I had it with me. How she grew and "enlarged the place of her tent" yet remained always *centered* in a demanding and illuminating faith in an order in the universe, in a *reason* for what seemed often in her private life like deprivation. She says it often:

> The truth is that solitude is the creative condition of genius, religious or secular, and the ultimate sterilizing of it. No human soul can for long ignore "the giant agony

of the world" and live except indeed the mollusc life, like a barricade upon eternity. (p. 297)

And later in a letter to her sister Meg:

Because if one loves, one really isn't lonely; it is the unloving heart that is always cold, and has no fire to warm itself at. "Beloved, let us love one another, for love is of God, and he that loveth is born of God *and knoweth God*". Don't tell me there are theological explanations of it—that the love must be "in Christ." He that loveth—knoweth God. Which means when the heart goes out to anything, it is, in that moment, close to God.

York Hospital, Monday, June 30

A BAD NIGHT, about three hours sleep because one hour after I was in deep sleep I was wrenched awake by a male nurse to take my blood pressure, etc. It was then eleven (a nurse had done it at nine-thirty). At one-fifteen I asked for another pill, maybe slept by three, and meanwhile went into a tailspin of depression. To manage such a passive *waiting* life for so many months I have had to bury my real self—and now realize that bringing that real self back is going to be even more difficult than it was to bury it. The fact is that in this state of accidie there is nothing I look forward to, no one I long to see or be with—Bramble haunted me and her loss came back with great poignance. With her death some secret wild place in me has gone. Shall I ever find it again?

The counterpoint for this time of negation and nothingness

has been the curious combination of an almost daily call from Pat Keen in Los Angeles with news of *Nicholas Nickleby*, which is having a great and deserved triumph there, and my call to Juliette Huxley. Juliette had the courage at eighty-nine to fly to Crete alone for two weeks. She came home to a heat wave in London! But the reviews of her splendid autobiography are good and she sounded very much on a wave of relief when I called her yesterday morning.

The contrast between these two friends, so much alike in the struggle, and my snail-like existence is ridiculous. I want to be well.

I note a typical hospital day which begins at:

    7:00 A.M. — male night nurse brings Metamucil and orange juice

    7:30 A.M. — brush teeth, nurse comes with pills and to take my temperature, etc.

    8:00 A.M. — breakfast

    8:25 A.M. — nurse to do a rhythm test of my heart

    8:30 A.M. — Edythe with the mail. Pat calls from L.A. while she is here, and when she leaves for a moment I let all the frustrations and grief out

    8:45 A.M. — a wheel chair to take me to Cardiology for an "echo" test

    9:15 A.M. — longing to get a snooze but it's time for a shower and the nurse makes my bed while I'm having it

    9:30–
10:30 A.M. — read the mail and papers

11:30 A.M. — Nancy comes

12 Noon — lunch

12:30 P.M. — Dr. Petrovich

  1:00 P.M. — maid to clean room, nurse for vital signs and pills

Finally from 1:30 to 3:00 go fast asleep and have a vivid
dream of Louise Bogan

3:00 P.M. — Gail, nurse, comes in to take vital signs
4:00 P.M. — Edythe with wonderful ice cream and we
have a little walk

Tuesday, July 1

HOME AGAIN. I feel disoriented, without an identity. What a
strange time this is, all told. Watering the flowers helped. I
think one trouble is that I feel disassociated from the garden.
Karen is doing such a good job, but it's not my garden these
days. I look and admire but am not *connected*.

I cooked the salmon for our supper. Edythe will stay over
this first night "at home." Salmon, mayonnaise, boiled potatoes, peas, and hot fudge sauce on vanilla ice cream. A feast,
as at the end I could not swallow the hospital food.

Wednesday, July 2

HEAVY PERSISTENT RAIN—and it is good to resume my old
pattern and routine—to make a small start at least at living
my real life again. Pierrot slept beside me, stretched out full
length and purring very loudly, and that was a help last night.

Now I look at the piles and piles of letters—and wonder—it's an insoluble problem at this point, so maybe just pull one or two out by chance.

I have nothing exhilarating to read at the moment. How impoverished a town York is without a single bookstore! There were two when I first came here. I'm feeling the emptiness of six months with almost no outside stimulation. I haven't been in a shop or bookstore all that time, or out to dinner except once, and have seen only my entourage of Nancy, Edythe and Janice—and Pat the two weeks she was here, in which I was, I'm afraid, mostly in a kind of trance—just trying to keep things going in the house. I do look back with joy on our good long talks at tea time.

Edith Kennedy, the most brilliant conversationalist I have known, used to talk about "the frame of reference." With most of my friends here, dear as they are, the frame of reference is very small in scope. When it suddenly widens what a joy it is! And I think back to such a moment when I had supper in New York with Marguerite and Jacques Barzun and we were talking of the Mozart film—and he and I leapt together remembering Yvonne Printemps in Sacha Guitry's delicious "Mozart" perhaps fifty years ago in Paris! What a bond to be with someone who remembered it and Printemps' aria:

> Si tu m'écris
> Dis-moi toujours que tu t'ennuies
> horriblement

Mozart sang it in farewell to three court ladies, each of whom might have been his mistress. But which one? That was the piquancy of the scene.

Pat is dear to me partly *because* the frame of reference between us is very wide. She has read enormously—and there is the theater, too—and Jung—and all that a European woman has in her blood.

Thursday, July 3

IT'S STILL GRAY, cold and miserable after yesterday's deluge and I feel tired and cross—bored by this half-life, and not quite ready, perhaps, for a full one.

Pierrot is proving to be a problem—using my bathroom mat at night although he has a pan in my bedroom close by. So I again threw the bath mat in the washer—and we shall see. This time I forced him to smell it and spanked him. Meanwhile Tamas, who is always so good, had had diarrhea in the night and there were *three* rugs to clean up downstairs!

But I'm determined to get something done at my desk, for morale's sake.

Friday, July 4

STATUE OF LIBERTY DAY! It has been quite a celebration and I feel proud this time of the media who really made an effort to talk about the hell Ellis Island was. We, my mother and I, came that way and she would never talk about it, she had been so terribly humiliated. The miracle is that the great waves of "foreigners"—Irish, Italians, Greeks, Jews—really have been assimilated. I must say, too, that in spite of my nostalgia for Europe I am glad to be an American. Among other good things, to write in English. But for World War I, I should have been a Belgian poet in a tiny country divided between two languages.

It's been a lovely quiet day; the only sound, the sea gulls crying and the murmur of ocean. I felt rather sick after lunch— dreading the return of that awful feeling from the drug, but maybe it will grow less—and maybe Dr. Petrovich will reduce the dose to one every other day. I think I can handle that.

I'm really getting ready for the fall trips—hoping against hope I shall be able to do them. Rather dismayed to find how far Burlington, Vermont, is—where I'm due September twenty-fourth for a reading. I had imagined Edythe might drive me there. But it looks as though I would have to take a plane from Boston.

Pierrot has been very affectionate all day and last night behaved himself, thank goodness. The great adventure was going for a walk. He bounds or rather tears after or ahead of us, then gets frightened and *wails* until I call him. When a motorcar passed us very slowly he was terrified and disappeared entirely. I called and called, heard no mews—and was quite anxious, but there he was waiting for us when we got home, Tamas and I.

I found a tick under my knee. They have been the worst ever this year, but had seemed to be over lately. How repulsive they are!

Saturday, July 5

AN IN AND OUT DAY—but there's no doubt that having to pull oneself together is a help. Heidi had agreed to meet me at Barnacle Billy's for lunch, so I had an incentive to get things done and did a laundry, swept the kitchen, took rubbish down cellar (luckily Raymond was here when I got back from lunch so it was all ready for him to take).

Sunday, July 6

HORRIBLE MUGGY GRAY DAY. I got up full of determination at five-thirty, let Tamas out, made bacon for Sunday breakfast for Tamas and me. Pierrot was out bird watching. After breakfast, put fresh sheets on my bed and washed and folded the dirty ones—and meanwhile had decided to make *ratatouille* before the ingredients Edythe got for me rotted. It took nearly an hour to cut everything up and get it started—so I can finish the cooking tonight now the work is done. All very well, but now it is nine forty-five and I am thinking of taking a nap instead of writing letters!

I had such a good talk with Carol on the phone just before six—she thinks I am right to go out and do poetry readings whatever the risk. That gave me a boost. I think she understands my slow starvation these past months and reading the poems will help give me back the person I have lost.

Carol was interesting about Frances Partridge—saying she was never the central person to *herself*—and that I have been that and am that. Yes, if I can write poetry again—ever again. For to be the central person for oneself implies that one is somehow the servant of something greater than oneself.

Wednesday, July 9

WELL, the old heart is out of sync, fibrillating and running about 140 a minute—so I'm back to square one and determined to get Dr. Petrovich to agree on the operation at Massachusetts General which would free me, I hope, from the long struggle.

We are having a heat wave, although today there is less humidity and it is quite bearable.

I must go back to Monday because I got back a little of the magic of this place when all was ready, champagne on ice, glasses, a plate of cookies, for Bill Heyen and Han and Bill Ewart who brought one of their boys. I sat down as I have not done lately, watching the light dancing in the leaves of the lilac, and feeling happy and at peace, glad that friends would soon be here. And such good friends. Bill Heyen is one of the very few poets I know now. I admire his work, tender, deep and authentic as it is, and I love him, great blond man. And of course Bill Ewart is the magician who imagines and prints the Christmas poem for me and once a little book of poems—and will do another tiny book next year. So all was festive for their arrival, even to a blue sea—and we had a good talk. I'm afraid Han, slight and shy, was disappointed in the garden—there is so little to see these days. But the Japanese iris are coming out!

And suddenly this afternoon a huge bunch of flame-colored roses arrived from Laurie Shields way off in San Francisco at the Older Women's League.

Bill's son, who has a sheltie, was dear with Tamas, stroking and talking to him just as though he were a person, as indeed he is.

Lucy just called from Dr. Petrovich's office—he is going to get hold of Dr. Ruskin, the "guru" for this operation, so at last I may get well soon! Unbelievable!

Friday, July 11

BUT NOW IT SEEMS Dr. Ruskin is away until the end of August—and Dr. P. is trying to get in touch with his assistant, Hasan Garan. I meanwhile feel awfully sick and abandoned this week end, still having to take the infernal medicine. And it is an almost perfect July day, warm and dry, the air so clear everything is in sharp outline.

How can I ever tell all the people who have sent flowers? Today a charming blue and white arrangement in a basket, very pale yellow lilies, iris, some little soft flowers in button-shaped branches that look like a wild flower, and harebells! The latter seem like magic in a florist's bouquet—this one from Dorothy Peck whom I have never met, but we talk occasionally on the phone.

Flowers and the telephone have kept me from despair. Jabber called from St. Louis yesterday. Pat Keen calls every morning from Los Angeles.

I have forgotten to speak of the good night sounds, the steady pulse of the crickets and gentle sea murmurs in the distance—and the other night I was kept awake by a mockingbird who sang the three songs he had learned without stopping from midnight to three! It was a mixed pleasure although one of the songs, a curious chuck-chuck between arias, reminded me of a nightingale.

[And where and when did I get to know the nightingale's song? At Grace Dudley's in Vouvray. Her house was called Le Petit Bois, and in that little wood we once walked out in moonlight and heard six nightingales. That was just after World War II in the forties, an eon ago.]

Wednesday, July 16

A LOT OF DAYS without a word here. The word would have been simply nausea, day after day, seven or eight hours of it, lying around waiting for the operation to be scheduled at Massachusetts General. They promise this *will* be done today. I can hardly wait as the possibility of feeling *well* again hovers in the air. Meanwhile it was a tremendous fillip to see Royce Roth and Frances Whitney, settled in at Dockside for their yearly holiday—my second dinner "out" in seven months. It was great fun and the good talk as always. I have been starved for that.

Now at last Lucy called and the Massachusetts General operation is scheduled for August third (my mother's birthday)—the seventeen days to wait feeling so ill really did come as a shock two hours ago. Now I have thought it over, I see that I must take it as a challenge, to use these days for some really life-enhancing things. It is a great help that Frances and Royce will be here the whole time. Maggie Vaughan will come Friday and bring our supper.

Thursday, July 17

NOW ALL THESE DAYS I am close to rage instead of tears, the two sides of depression, but rage may be healthier.

I feel sad that Pierrot is such a selfish, greedy cat—beautiful, of course, but a little affection would go a long way. Last night when I was pretty desperate and also exhausted by all the calls I had had to make, he never even came upstairs. He is heavy for me to carry up and sometimes he does come.

I am reading Peter Taylor's stories. He is compared to Chekhov on the jacket; in a way it is the same meager and comfortless, in a spiritual sense, life that is depicted, but C. is shot through with compassion. I think also about a lot of things that never get into this journal. Why? Because of the letters, a vast chaotic heap. Why? Because I do not have the psychic energy to write with any pith. And that is why I feel I have lost control of my life, look forward to *nothing*, live the days through like a zombi, and long for sleep, oblivion.

Saturday, July 19

FRIENDS, true friends, are life savers. Maggie Vaughan came yesterday, looking lovely and summery in a dress with a lily of the valley pattern—and as always laden with dear home-made things: a dozen fresh eggs, three small veal meat loaves, spinach from the garden, heavy cream from her Jersey cow, eggs in aspic for my lunches, raspberries for dessert and a whole set of plastic envelopes full of thin delicious cookies. I had felt rather sick all day, but just seeing Maggie's bright eyes and all those loving provisions revived me.

For once it was a gentle July evening with a little breeze to keep the mosquitoes away, and we sat out on the terrace and had ginger ale and cookies with Tamas, of course, eager for all the cookies he could wheedle, and Pierrot emerging from and disappearing into the bushes like a genie.

It is such a soothing open-ended way to talk, to be out-doors, yet sheltered, with the great ocean out there and an occasional yawl floating by. So Maggie and I caught up with ourselves. She is working with Hospice in Augusta and has been taking a course to that end.

After a while we went in to have a Scotch and look at the news—and have our wonderful supper. What Maggie had in mind was to recreate the *pain de veau* I mention in a chapter of *I Knew A Phoenix*, the *pain de veau* my father remem-bered and Maggie's creation was absolutely delicious and must have been an exact replica, in my view perhaps even better.

Today it is foggy and rainy and I felt so tired I got up late, but Maggie sat on the end of my bed with her coffee and we talked in a homey way.

Sunday, July 20

I GUESS THE FAST HEARTBEAT inevitably makes me feel tired all the time—so everything is an effort in the morning—again cold and gray—there seemed little motivation to get up at all. What pulled me up finally at nearly seven—I had let Tamas out at five-thirty—was knowing that Pierrot must be waiting outside, hoping for breakfast to appear—and there he was. Then I did a wash of shirts, pajamas and such, and had a bath. Now I have just called Juliette Huxley in London to catch up with her. She had been for a long walk on the Heath. How nostalgic I felt hearing that—and that at nearly ninety she can do it! Whereas I can walk only a few yards without losing my breath. It is now fourteen days to what I hope will be my emancipation.

I forgot to note here the marvelous changes outside: now the field is a strange pinkish color, the tall grasses ripple in the wind, and the thread of the path through it is bright emerald green. It is more than six months since I have walked down to the sea but I listen to it more than ever, great presence that is never still.

I also forgot to note how much I enjoy my daily drive to the post office, about four miles, first through the woods on this place, then out to salt marshes, and there I watch every day for a small inlet where two geese, two brown ducks and

a white one swim about together. If I see them my heart leaps
up and I feel happy—and can't help saying what I remember
of William Allingham's:

> Four ducks on a pond,
> A grass-bank beyond,
> A blue sky of spring,
> White clouds on the wing:
> What a little thing
> To remember for years,—
> To remember with tears!*

Later on, once in town, I observe the very few cared-for
small gardens and what is blooming there. Here the only
glorious thing to see is New Dawn, a cascade these days of
pale pink roses over the fence—at least they have flourished
in this summer when nothing else has.

Monday, July 21

DRIVING SLOWLY to pick up Royce and Frances last evening,
I looked at all the wild flowers along the road, the summer
crop just coming into bloom—meadow rue, goldenrod, herb
willow—their names taste of summer days and evenings. I
had felt really ill all day, but so looked forward to what we
had imagined would be a gala dinner at Arrows, one of the
few Maine restaurants in *Gourmet*, Royce said. We had been
there before, enjoying sitting in the wide porch looking out

---

* In *Come Hither*, comp. by Walter de la Mare (Knopf, 1960), p. 517.

on a garden. But it has changed hands—the *maitre d'* a young man in open shirt and trousers, very casual, said he had no note of a reservation for Roth, though Royce had called the day before. He was so high and mighty that we were tempted to leave, but he finally deigned to seat us and then we were confronted with a ridiculously expensive menu—that we suspected would not be worth the fortune involved. Quite right.

But we had a wonderful talk, partly about what the perfect marriage is if there is such a thing, and all agreeing that the end is friendship, the desideratum, it must begin and end there. Any such talk always sends me back to Homer as quoted by Vita Sackville-West and Harold Nicolson in their anthology *Another World Than This*:

> For there is nothing more potent or better than this: when a man and a woman, sharing the same ideas about life, keep house together. It is a thing which causes pain to their enemies and pleasure to their friends, but only they themselves know what it really means.

Wednesday, July 23

YESTERDAY I FELT so ill I almost called off lunch with Huldah who drove over from Center Sandwich. Today I have written a few letters and set the table very happily for Anne and Barbara, and feel better. I saw Lucy, Dr. Petrovich's assistant, yesterday afternoon, and much to my amazement the EKG showed a perfectly synchronized heartbeat which she attributes to the medicine—Amiodoroni—which has to accumulate in the system to do its work. Terrified that Dr. Petrovich will now want me to cancel the operation, I insisted that my heart might be normal but my intestinal tract was not. For I could not undertake a lecture trip in my present state. Also Lucy thinks the irregular heartbeat will slide in and out, no certainty that it will stay normal.

A perfect summer day here—the ocean absolutely calm, that Fra Angelico blue with a lighter band all along the horizon.

It was good to see Huldah after more than a year, looking just the same, although her deafness is a problem. But we had a really good "catching up" talk, nevertheless.

When we came back here there was a tiny exquisite mouse sitting on the rug in the porch—Pierrot was out. I screamed for help and Huldah, after several tries, managed to capture it in a paper towel and took it far off in the garden, near Bramble's tombstone. Pierrot must have brought it in alive earlier on. Will it live after such trauma?

I love mice but it is the sudden motions, the fear of picking it up, that scares me so. I was awfully grateful for Huldah's help.

She is very good—in Brentwood, Tennessee, too—about feeding household scraps to wild animals and told me she is now feeding a small fox and has seen him. I have not seen a fox here for a long time. There is so much building going on, the wilderness, here as everywhere, is literally losing ground. There are fewer birds also, no grosbeak this year at the feeder.

Friday, July 25

I LAY IN Dr. Petrovich's office in a johnny for forty-five minutes yesterday afternoon, waiting and crying with fear and tension. He finally got there. I said firmly, "I have two possibilities, the operation or suicide, for I can't go on feeling so ill, unable to work." He *still* asked if I had not felt better since Tuesday—when the heart began a normal beat—but Tuesday was the worst day for nausea in a long time. Then, the bombshell, "They may refuse to do the operation if your heart is normal when you go on August third. They are academics," he said, "you have to realize that." So I go in to Boston on August third and may be sent right back here! It is so preposterous after this long agonized wait that the only thing to do is curl up inside and sit it out.

Monday, July 28

WHERE HAVE THE DAYS since Friday gone? Very depressing, foggy, humid awful weather for one reason, plus the fact that I feel worse rather than better and have a dull pain in my heart all the time—worse nausea than before. But Saturday morning I had the great joy of seeing Susan Garrett who came

with strawberries to sit down and catch up a little, especially
on my problems lately. She is such a sensitive, compassionate
person. How I wish she were still director of the hospital
here! But of course George is a professor at Charlottesville
and they are here to inhabit her father's dear old house on
the river only for a few summer days. Seeing Susan was like
an infusion of love and caring. "A *piqûre*," Edith Kennedy
used to call that.

That afternoon Royce and Frances for champagne—and
in all the heavy heat there came a saving waft of air from the
ocean and we sat outside for a while, then inside, for some
reason got off on a passionate political argument, and I felt
ill when they left after only a little more than an hour and
could not eat anything. That meant that Pierrot and Tamas
had a feast—the half-cold tenderloin steak!

Yesterday I again felt too sick to look forward to the real
event of Eleanor Blair's coming with Elyce, bringing our lunch.
I haven't been able to get over to Eleanor since before Christmas. What a joy to see her, blooming at ninety-one, having
recovered from a broken wrist in record time, and lit up by
Elyce's presence as she always is. Elyce teaches economics
at the University of Indiana—where I'm supposed to be October 13–18, God willing—and knows Eleanor because she
was her tenant on an exchange year at Wellesley. It has turned
into a remarkable friendship.

She had made a fruit salad and a special yogurt and mango
sauce—and luckily I had put a bottle of Vouvray in the fridge
which tasted perfect with the fruit and the Brie.

I was amazed at how much Eleanor was able to see although she is legally blind. She noticed all the changes in the
library due to the fire and remembered the little ring of Net-
suke round a bowl of shells, for instance. How can she see
them, I wonder?

Elyce meanwhile was fascinated by Pierrot in one of his

wilder moods—what dismay when I found earlier that day an awful mess he had made in the corner of the library! I heard him scratching and rushed in—oh dear! I wish he would learn that the whole great outdoors is there for his purposes!

I wish I had something long, absorbing and rich to read! I have ordered Yeats' letters but they haven't come, but it adds to my feeling of being in limbo not to have anything to read. I thought I would reread V. Woolf's *The Years*, but found it too depressing—the too vivid account at first of the household where the wife and mother is dying upstairs—not what I need right now.

Today a last meeting with Fran and Royce who leave on Wednesday and are coming to take me out to lunch. I'm glad to get away. My desk is a nightmare of the undone and will stay like that unless I can be well and write ten or twenty letters a day as I sometimes did on the week ends.

Tuesday, July 29

HARD TO SAY GOOD-BY to Royce and Fran. When I got up from my nap around four I began to cry and couldn't stop. I feel as ill or worse than ever—with the fear hanging over me that they will refuse to do the operation because my heart is—or was last week—in sync, due to the medicine. It is too ironic!

Dr. Petrovich has doubled my dose of Bumex because I pant so much.

But I did pick a funny little bunch of flowers for the house in the late afternoon: self-sown nicotiana, opium poppies, veronica, day lilies, Shasta daisies, "an artless bouquet" as the interviewer from the *Times* described my indoor flowers— but it was a real pleasure to do it and I must tell Karen so. She has soldiered on without enough interest or praise from me, I know, and she is so dear with Tamas, he will miss her. I shall feel forlorn when she goes back to Tucson on August fifteenth.

Thursday, July 31

I LAY AWAKE a long time last night listening to the rain, and thought how badly I have handled myself lately. Loneliness has taken over what used to be a vitalizing solitude, a pause between poetry readings and seeing many friends who used to come. Now I feel abandoned and desolate—and would like to miaow in the way Pierrot does now and then to say, "Where are you? I'm lonely!"

People, especially Janice, with all her nursing knowledge and compassionate spirit, have been as supportive as they could. But Anne and Barbara are far away—everyone after all has someone important, a job—I become the extra effort in their full-to-capacity lives. And so, I must admit, I have been for years myself, the quick responder to cries of help, often from people I have never seen, but who write to me as a friend. One reason for my depression now is that I can no longer "respond" as I used to. I feel so cut off from what was once a self.

Everyone I know must be as sick and tired of this illness as I am.

People, friends, do come, and Nancy's daily arrival at eight all week is of immeasurable comfort. She is so steady and so kind, it is a blessing—and she is very good to Tamas and the Wild Beast, Pierrot, too. On the days when she is not here, a sort of blackness takes over the house and me.

Of course what is lacking is the tangible "we" when two people live together in amity—and at seventy-four I have to admit that the likelihood of its ever happening again is slight.

In spite of the gloom yesterday I made brownies, so all is not lost!

Friday, August 1

BACK FROM LUNCH with Edythe to find a note from Nancy to say "prepare to be admitted to Phillips House on Saturday." I called them of course. "Why?" "Because otherwise you might not get a room." They will call me between nine and eleven Saturday morning and I won't know till then. I felt dizzy.

[For one thing the Molnar-Fentons were supposed to be coming Saturday afternoon to be shown around as I am lending them the house for a holiday while I'm away. Dorothy Molnar and Stephen Fenton came to see me six or seven years ago because, they told me, it was reading my poems that had brought them together and so I was a kind of godmother to their marriage. They were at that time social workers and I was drawn to them both. Dorothy's oval face and blue eyes reminded me of my mother's, and Stephen's black beard and rosy cheeks, his bright eyes full of tenderness, charmed me.

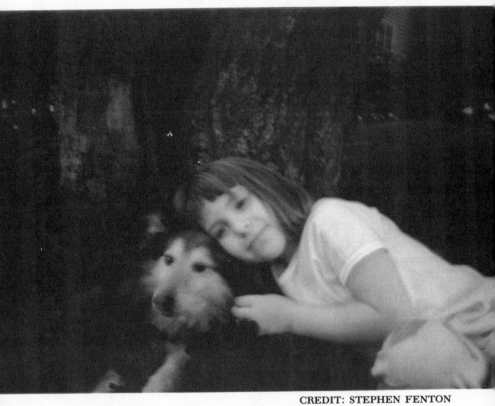

Little Sarton with Tamas

So I was deeply touched when two years later I had the announcement of the birth of their first child and saw that she had been named for me, her first name "Sarton."

Last summer they all three spent a vacation in Ogunquit so I saw something of them and they began to feel like family. When I picked them up at Foster's, little Sarton, now five, was happy to ride with me. She said, "It is very hard to be five. So much is expected of you," and I was delighted as I think everyone feels this about whatever age he or she may be. Sarton is a ravishing little girl with a Dutch cut that reminds me of myself at her age and wide-apart blue eyes. She observes everything and, of course, Tamas is in his element and adores any little girl not much taller than he.

So I had offered to lend them the house this summer. I had planned to go to the Cape to Rene Morgan's that week when the Massachusetts General Hospital intervened. Because I could not show them the house I worked hard putting labels on all the drawers and cupboards to say where things were in the kitchen. Then all Saturday morning I waited for a call while Edythe Haddaway and her friend, Betty, waited to be told to come and fetch me. Finally at eleven I called. A new crew takes over on the week end. They had no message for me. "You are booked for Sunday at one-thirty," I was told. All that suspense, all the frantic arrangements, the Molnar-Fentons put off, Edythe and Betty put off. It made me furious. I had so looked forward to seeing little Sarton before I left, and making the house feel like a good nest for them, all three.

Dorothy was wonderful on the phone. They will just walk in here at noon on Sunday after I leave and will spend tonight at a motel in Ogunquit. The logistics of all this made me so agitated I felt terribly sick all that afternoon.] As Dorothy compassionately put it, "Nothing goes smoothly for you these days."

Phillips House, Massachusetts General Hospital, Boston, Monday, August 4

I KNOW NOW what it must be like to be a dog in a cage not knowing why it is there—hoping, waiting, punished she doesn't know why or what for—for I lay in a cubicle in the Emergency ward—I had been called at ten and told to go there and be admitted—from one-fifteen to six forty-five—lying with a heart monitor on behind me so I could not move or get up. After four hours I asked to be allowed to go to the bathroom. "A bedpan is all we can offer," said a sadistic nurse who was as mean as they come. I explained that I found it hard to function that way and she sneered, "Well, you'll come to it." Finally a black male nurse got me out of my misery by breaking the rules, and let me into the nurses' toilet. Relief! I had had breakfast at six, but when the head nurse offered to bring food I knew I couldn't eat it. Three doctors took my history. One, a handsome young man, must have passed by me through the room a hundred times in those interminable hours but never smiled or said, "Hang in there." When I complained about the long wait, a nurse said, "You are lucky. Some people wait twenty-four hours." Whenever I asked, "Has Phillips House been notified?" the head nurse said, more than once, "Yes." But when Maggie came at five she was told I was not in the hospital!

Phillips House, Wednesday, August 6

I HAVE BECOME acclimatized to hospital life, I think, and am no longer a trapped hedgehog with all its bristles erect. There have been a lot of tests, as I expected. I had a very good talk with the surgeon on Monday, and he talked in terms of the operation and pacemaker, but that afternoon I was brought a pill, a drug that has not been tried in York, called verapamil hydrochloride, taken three times a day, and my heart sank. No operation after all? I burst into tears.

Maggie Vaughan, the dear woman, is staying at the Holiday Inn during these days to be my support—comes twice a day—brought delicious gingerbread with her which greatly improves jello as a dessert—and ginger ale. She leaves today.

I am awfully homesick now and tired of the deadly hospital atmosphere, bland at best, cold and inhuman at worst.

Pat Keen arrives Sunday.

I have wonderful flowers—from friends near and far. After the traumatic hours of admission, I found a lavender freesia plant from Vicky Simon, such an intimate *real* thing to find in an impersonal room!

J. T. and Cora sent flowers—a marvelous variety all different colors like some dream of flowers—in the center a red and white lily, then pink African daisies, a deep purple flower that looks like a poppy—it is Japanese—those South American small lilies in a very bright orange—more than I can name.

Polly Starr delivered a rainbow of gladiola from her garden in Hingham: pink, lavender, orange—a clap of cymbals.

Judy Burrowes sent an exquisite basket all blues and whites: freesia, white snapdragons, delphinium.

And there were heartening phone calls from R.H.C. in Oregon, from Charles Feldstein, my adopted brother in Chicago, from Pat in Los Angeles, Rene Morgan on the Cape, as well as from friends nearer by.

And I hear the news from home every day from Dorothy and hold in my heart the treasure that she and Stephen and little Sarton are having marvelous days—as is Tamas who goes on long walks with them. Pierrot did not come in Sunday night—he is very shy and easily frightened—but has now decided that all is well and has become part of the family.

Hospital hilarity: a woman just came in and asked, "Would you like to do any needlework?" Since it is difficult for me to sew on a button it made me laugh.

I have been reading Mary Gordon's *Men and Angels*, which I found repulsive at first but am now absorbed in, and yesterday Maggie brought me *The Hospice Movement*, which will be real nourishment, I know.

My friends have surrounded me with love—and that should make me well. I forgot to say that among the phone calls have been two from Fred Rogers—"Mr. Rogers"—the dear man. I could hardly believe my ears. He is off to Nantucket—how glad I was to know he would get some rest though he said, "I have to do some writing."

Phillips House, Thursday, August 7

I CAN GO HOME TOMORROW but hope to wait till Saturday so Sarton's holiday will not be cut short. Dr. Garan came in around six—just as my dinner was brought in—to explain *why* the operation and pacemaker have been decided against. My heart has been shown to be weaker than they knew or expected—and what is weak is the atrium's electrical stimulus which sends blood into the ventrical. The pacemaker *only* affects the ventrical, so would or might only do harm. "The operation is irreversible," he said. But he also said *if* I had heart failure, which could happen, they would then as a last resort do the operation! He said, "By all means go on your lecture tour," and is confident the pill will work. I'll still have to take Coumadin and do the blood test for that maybe every two weeks. So I'm really back at square one and not sorry to be—*if* this pill works.

[I got into a panic at first because I began to have those cramps again, and when I met Dr. Kelly in the hall, asked if I could see her for a minute. "I am very busy," she said and walked away. Then followed me to the desk and asked in an irritated voice, "What is the matter?" I murmured that I was afraid the old symptoms were coming back and the pill might not work, a natural enough fear under the circumstances. "You were perfectly all right yesterday," she said and turned on her heel.

Now that Dr. Garan has made his decision I can see I am to be ignored. They are through with me.]

I want to end this episode of the hospital with these pertinent remarks from *The Hospice Movement*:

> It is a strange embrace we now find welcoming us into the place called *hospital*. It is one which neutralizes instantly whatever life force it is that makes each one of us into a unique individual. *Hospital* welcomes my body as so many pounds of meat, filled with potentially interesting mechanical parts and neurochemical combinations. *Hospital* strips one of all personal privacy, of all sensual pleasure, of every joy the flesh finds delight in; and at the same time, seizes me in a total embrace. *Hospital* makes war, not love.

I must believe that I am going home to be *well*, to find myself again, to function as my *self*.

Saturday, August 9

I WAS MOVED the last night into a cell-like room at Baker— no one told me I could turn on the television by paying three dollars. It would have been well worth it. No towels. No light over the bed. But the nurses I saw were all very kind—one even recognized my name. I was to leave at ten. They forgot my breakfast. Edythe came at nine-thirty and we got a cart so she could wheel down the flowers I had chosen from the many in the other room and my suitcase and briefcase and pack Betty's car where Betty waited—and waited—and waited. Dr. Kelly only got to me with the prescriptions at eleven-fifteen! The thing that saved me that last night was reading

the Hospice book which Maggie brought. It took me right
out of self-pity and ugly surroundings to pure love.

In the hospital I had dreamed of home and saw it all as a
dream, composed and quiet, full of beauty and the eternal
murmur of the ocean, but when I got back after lunch and
was alone here, the house fell on my shoulders like a heavy
weight. All there is to do! For Pat arrives tomorrow night.

Pierrot recognized me and purred when I picked him up,
but Tamas does not like the bed I had ordered from L. L.
Bean's with so much joy. It is too big for him and I must
change it for a smaller one. At last nasturtiums are out in the
garden.

Sunday, August 10

A FINE SUMMER DAY and no thunderstorms for a change! I've
accomplished quite a lot—mostly dragging in food—how heavy
melons are! It took one hour and a half—partly because of
getting crabmeat—for I have invited Karen Olch and her friend
for lunch tomorrow. The fish market is in the center of York
Beach and it took me over half an hour of stop-and-go along
the beach itself. How inviting the water looked, lovely little
waves ruffling the edge of the ocean and people looking happy.

Monday, August 11

WHEN I SAT DOWN to look at the news, with macaroni and cheese in the oven, I found the television was not working! Finally I got through to the right number and a very kind young man drove up in about an hour, climbed a tree with a ladder and fixed whatever it was. Pat got here in the warm summer night around quarter past nine—and it was good to see her. How thankful I am to Edythe for meeting the plane, which was an hour late!

It rained in the night and will be hot and steamy for sure. The crabmeat salad is all made and the chicken stuffed for tonight, so I am on my way "with miles to go before I sleep." I am tired, but able to cope—that is the good news. Hurrah!

Tuesday, August 12

AMAZING—I can hardly take in that I do feel better, that I am myself again. I am so happy I managed to have Karen Olch and her friend for lunch and was able, I think, to tell Karen what she has done for me this summer, and under the difficult circumstances that I was not really here in spirit to see what she had done and appreciate it fully. I needed to say this and to thank her properly. The last two weeks since Debby arrived from Tucson have been too backed up, too much to do, too many people to say good-by to, so she is at the raw edge of exhaustion—and it showed when she came here to work. In the early days she was so happy to be here, so dear with Tamas, she seemed glowing with the pleasure of it and worked like a beaver. She is a brave woman, one of five who burst through police to pour ashes on the memorial, a bronze replica of a nuclear mushroom, at Pease Air Force Base on the anniversary of Hiroshima. They were arrested, then the case held off for weeks. I think they got community work as penalty and she will be allowed to do it in Tucson.

After Karen and Debby left I washed the dishes, tidied up and had a nap, or rested, till half past three, time to get the chicken out and light the oven. Later Pat and I had a wonderful peaceful hour on the terrace watching the sunset at the back of the house reflected on the ocean and in the sky. It had been dark blue in the late afternoon, then became absolutely calm like pale blue satin, with a dark line at the horizon which Pat noted made it look like a Japanese print. Finally the clouds took on a rosy glow and the sea became *pink*.

After supper and in bed at about ten, I heard an owl hooting repeatedly—and finally answered by another owl. I woke Pat up to hear it. Before this she had tried to track down Pierrot with a flashlight. Elusive creature, he loves to be chased and hates to be caught. I went down at ten and called, and then he did come in and ran right upstairs to my bed— but it was hot and he did not stay. The floor is best for him when it is over eighty, but the night was pleasantly cool by the time I got to sleep.

Wednesday, August 13

PAT IS A TREMENDOUS HELP this time—sees things that need to be done and does them, and we are having a peaceful, talkative, homey time as I had hoped we might. From her room the raccoon's mischievous attacks on the bird feeders are only too audible—the wire clatters and bangs.

We sat on the terrace earlier on and had tea but Raymond, suddenly assiduous, drove up with his lawn mower which he said did not work after all—so typical—but then he stood beside us and we talked of this and that for a half hour. He looks diminished and much older these days. I am the more grateful that Diane York, a friend of Karen's who lives in Kittery, will come early Friday morning to take the rubbish— and Raymond will be released at last. She will start work soon on the invasion of wild blackberry that is getting serious among the daffodils.

Yesterday I began to work on the poem for Bramble. I felt it would be the test and prove I was well—and I have worked on it again today and—glory be!—played music, two Mozart concerti.

Thursday, August 14

THE BEAUTIFUL WEATHER HOLDS cool and bright with a little breeze in the evening. I am so happy for Pat. The only misery is her having been terribly bitten by mosquitoes when she lay out on the terrace day before yesterday and was *devoured*.

We are having lunch with Nancy and Edythe at the York Harbor Inn, and I go to the hairdresser for the first time in two weeks this morning, so time is running away at a fast clip! Eleanor will be here cleaning soon—it is just after nine now.

I am exhilarated by the decision to go on the lecture tour— that rapid descent into real old age has been stopped. And I am going to be all right—after all I felt very unwell all last fall on the road and that was a triumphal tour. The only bother is clothes—but I have enough. I'll manage.

Pat amazes and delights me with all her talents—she has three pianos in her flat in Ipswich, and brought her flute and also painting materials with her. How slowly one gets really to know someone, but now I feel we are building a solid foundation. It is a treat for me to be with someone who has read so much—thought so much, too. And, of course, in a strange way we meet on European ground.

Jean Dominique's birthday today—how long since she died? And hardly a day passes that I do not think of her. [And as I think of her I often think of "La Petite Espérance" which Péguy speaks of, and which is so hard to translate. I went back to an essay Jean Dominique wrote for the Brussels *Soir* in 1939 to find exactly what Péguy had said and what Jean-Do had said.

The great tremor of our souls and of our thoughts has been bathed this year as in 1914 in an ideal season. A pure warm sky has shed on the first days of September an abundant peaceful light which resembled—anguished though hearts were—an immense banner of profound hope. Instinctively, eyes that looked for signs, as they looked out on the thick leaves over gardens and avenues, began to count the invincible reasons that man has to honor life by a happy impulse of his whole being. The majesty of trees became a lesson in confidence and balance, as did the elastic resistance of grass, or the trembling attempt at flying of late butterflies chasing each other above the phlox . . .

Nevertheless more than ever before we must sustain that hope, and we verify at every moment that it is for Péguy (and for God himself when Péguy listens to him speak) the most beautiful, the most necessary, the hardest of virtues.

"I am," says God, "the Lord of that virtue.

"Faith is a great tree. It is an oak rooted in the heart of France. And under the wings of that tree, Charity, my daughter, shelters all the pain in the world.

"But my little Hope

"Is she who every day

"Greets us with a good morning . . .

"Faith is a cathedral rooted in the heart of France.

"Charity is a hospital which picks up all the misery in the world.

"But without Hope, all that would be only a cemetery.

"My little Hope is she who goes to bed every night.

"And gets up every morning.

"And has really very good nights.

"I am, says God, the Lord of that virtue."

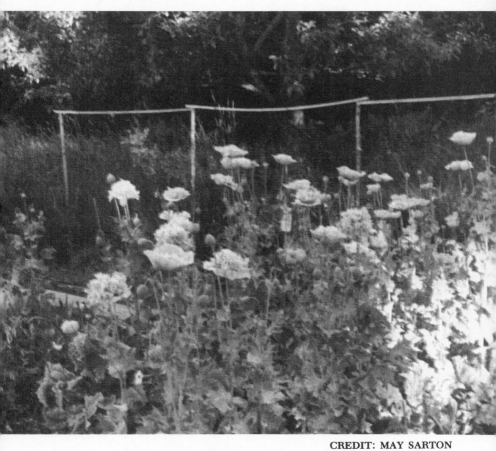

"opium poppies in their pink ruffles"

When my Dutch friend Hannie Van Till was in a Japanese prison camp in Java for four years, with ten thousand women, she told me that if they had known it would be four years they could not have survived. Hope kept them alive.]

Friday, August 15

TODAY is little Sarton's sixth birthday—so life goes on. I can hardly believe that I am well, went down through the wet grasses to pick a few nasturtiums for Pat. This is the first year they are plentiful and I feel sure it is Karen's feeding of them that did it. Calendulas are out, a very few small zinnias, a few bachelor's-buttons—only the self-sown nicotiana and opium poppies in their pink ruffles are really flourishing this bad summer for flowers. But at last there is something to pick and someone to pick for. I was too ill even to go down there for months.

Saturday, August 16

ANNE WOODSON called yesterday to tell me there was an obituary about Robbins Milbank in the *Globe*. I feel an awful pang that that sensitive and committed man is no longer on earth. It brings back such vivid memories of Nelson, of dinner with Helen and Robbins, and a wonderful picnic by the lake with Julia and Paul Child.

Pat left after lunch, managing somehow to carry her heavy bags to Edythe's little car in a misty rain. It gave me a strange feeling to walk back into the empty house—but we had good days and I do feel so much better it is marvelous. I am putting on my life again like a dear old corduroy jacket, worn but comfortable. It has been such an *un*comfortable life lately.

Sunday, August 17

OH DEAR it is now half past nine, so I think I must try to get up at five again instead of six. But it was such a joy to go down into the picking garden and pick a bunch of nasturtiums, then a great white lily and a few vermilion snapdragons to put around it—and nicotiana to freshen up a bouquet, and a whole bunch of calendulas, some pale orange, some with green hearts—at last they are doing well.

Before that I had washed my sheets, put on fresh ones, put away the dishes from the dishwasher—oh, and filled the bird feeders. The raccoon had pulled down the huge one, but I managed to fill and hang it, something I could not have done a month ago.

And now I am at my desk at last—looking out on a whitish ocean, which means hot humid air.

Pat called from New York so the little thread is there between us again—and all is well here for a change! All except the rapidity with which time flows away!

Monday, August 18

SUCH A HEAVY HUMID DAY I decided to run into Portsmouth to get a new blotter and pad for under the typewriter—and birdseed—now thirty-seven dollars for fifty pounds of hearts of sunflower! But they last longer and do not make a mess as sunflower seed does. I enjoyed the trip, but of course *not* writing letters after nine-thirty this morning simply adds to the mountain at my left.

I got Xeroxes of the fall poetry tour—it looks fun and not too tiring—and had a few copies made of my poem for Bramble too. It is still not *quite* right. But when I put on a Mozart concerto and wrote it last week, even though it is not good *enough*, I knew I was well at last.

With the grasses all golden now, the path through the field is a bright green ribbon as it winds down to the sea.

Tuesday, August 19

BEFORE I GO TO SLEEP, old forgotten poems often come to mind, this one by James Stephens in *Kings And the Moon* for instance. I had forgotten his charming inscription and was happy to find it again. This poem, "Tanist," comes back to me now because I have been struggling with a new problem. I used to be able to give lots of money away—the needs are everywhere. But as everyone insists that I do, illness has made me face the fact that I have what I earn plus social security— and a small income from the Shawmut Trust, not enough to live as I do and feel able to give large amounts away to individuals. So I have to deny myself generosity and sharply curb the galloping horse. This poem haunts me as it always has for we never do enough.

Remember the spider
Weaving a snare
—And that you did it
Everywhere:

Remember the Cat
Tormenting a bird
—And that you did it
In deed and word:

Remember the fool
Frustrating the good
—And that you did it
Whenever you could:

Remember the devil
And treachery
—And that you did it
When you were he:

Remember all ill
That men can know
—And that you did it
When you were so:

And then remember
Not to forget,
—That you did it
And do it yet.

A poem with great weaknesses, yet it has haunted me—at least it stabs smugness to the heart.

Another muggy day but the LeShans are coming at five to take me out to dinner—and that is a rare event.

Also Hurricane Charley has blown out to sea.

Wednesday, August 20

A WONDERFUL DAY YESTERDAY because Eda and Larry LeShan drove up from New York to celebrate with me their forty-second wedding anniversary! I didn't know what the occasion was except that they had been concerned about my health and we have not seen each other for a year, but I was touched when I heard what day it was for them. Luckily I had put a bottle of champagne on ice.

Larry had a severe heart attack in the spring, so we talked quite a lot about hospitals and he insisted that I write to the director of Massachusetts General—which I must do for the sake of others who have suffered as I did. Annella Brown called the other day and told me that a friend of hers had been kept in Emergency for six hours, sitting on a hard bench. It seems unbelievable.

Larry looks extremely well and is determined to smoke his pipe again soon. In the course of our conversation Eda said that when there was a certain kind of silence in the apartment, she knew Larry was reading my journals, which he has read and reread. "They give me peace," he said. Other people have said so, but his praise means a great deal—and so much for those who think of me as a writer pleasing only women!

They were very kind to Tamas who revels in attention and when he gets it almost becomes his old self again. Meanwhile Pierrot had disappeared—he had followed me down to the picking garden at around four and didn't come back, but thank goodness I did hear a mew at the door and knew he was safe before we left to have dinner at Dockside.

We sat at a splendid table in the window looking out at the harbor and off to the side so it was not noisy. I had a simply delicious sole stuffed with lobster. Eda had her ritualistic Maine lobster and Larry had a seafood mixture. This was followed—except for Larry whose doctor insists that he lose weight—by praline and walnut ice cream pie. Wow!

This morning Tamas managed the stairs so I shared my breakfast with him. It is the only intimate time together now and I treasure it. Pierrot displaces a great deal of atmosphere and comes to lie beside me at night—but I miss dear Tamas. I had to give up coaxing and laboring to get him upstairs at night when I was ill, and this is one of the real losses of old age as he and I grow old together. He is very lame these days.

The LeShans must be about ten years younger than I, so I felt rather proud to be myself and nearly seventy-five.

People imagine my life here as peaceful and sedentary, but they can't imagine of course what human problems pour in here every day. Yesterday a parcel which contained a letter and a cassette. An aunt whose nephew is dying of AIDS begged me to listen to the cassette, a concert which included his setting of two poems of mine—and to write him. I'll do that today.

A long unhappy letter from an old lady shut up in a nursing home—we have corresponded for years, and whatever else I don't do, I must write to her.

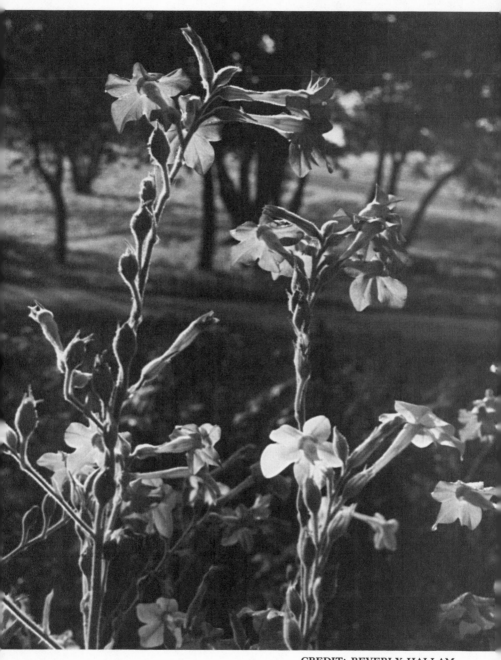

CREDIT: BEVERLY HALLAM

"self-sown nicotiana"

Thursday, August 21

YESTERDAY WAS perfect, clear and cool, and again today everything shines and sparkles with just a hint of autumn in the air. I went out to the garden and worked for a happy hour, cutting back the autumn-flowering clematis which had taken over half the fence, smothering the larger and more beautiful clematis that flower in June. Of course I am discovering all the things Karen did not have time to do. The lilies are doing very well; they had to be staked with longer stakes. It does seem very odd that the picking garden is finally, in late August, giving me flowers. Next year I'll buy more flats as the snapdragons I bought in flats are at present "best" of the lot. As usual self-sown nicotiana has taken over flower beds and must now be pulled out. The calendulas are delightful. I love the silky orange ones with green hearts.

It is impossible to write letters morning *and* afternoon, so I have decided to get back to my old routine of gardening in the afternoon—a way of rinsing my eye and feeling whole again. It is hard to say how tired I am of responding by letter, even to dear friends. The endless answering was always a problem, but now with diminishing energy—I have to remind myself that I *am* nearly seventy-five—it often seems beyond my strength and will.

I love writing to Juliette, but she is really the only correspondent I look forward to answering.

Friday, August 22

BECAUSE I AM WELL I no longer suffer from the acute loneliness I felt all spring and summer until now. Loneliness because in spite of all the kindnesses and concern of so many
friends there was no one who could fill the hole at the center
of my being—only myself could fill it by becoming whole
again. It was loneliness in essence for the *self*. Now that I can
work, taking up the healthy rhythm of the days, I am not at
all lonely. It means not writing letters in the afternoon but
going out-of-doors to the garden, and having a bath when I
come in, dirty and somehow relieved, as though the chaos
here in my study had fallen into place and it did not matter
too much that so many people have been left unanswered.

Yesterday I pulled out a lot of the nicotiana and the big
opium poppies—which have sown themselves here every
summer—so the garden, which was being smothered, has
some neat borders of flowers again. Imagine waiting for annuals till late August!

It is, I realized suddenly, my eye that suffers from disorder
and lack of form, so giving the garden some form again was
deeply satisfying whereas the untidy drawers and cupboards
do not really bother me, because they do not disturb the eye,
and only occasionally the back of my mind.

When I was ill I resented that I had some years ago called
old age an "ascension" in an essay which appeared on the Op
Ed page in the *Times*. It did seem too ironic for words, but
I believe there is some truth in it as I go back to it now. The

ascension is possible when all that has to be given up can be *gladly* given up—because other things have become more important. I panted halfway up the stairs, but I also was able to sit and watch light change in the porch for an hour and be truly attentive to it, not plagued by what I "ought" to be doing.

But the body is part of our identity, and its afflictions and discontents, its donkey-like refusal to do what "ought" to be done, destroys self-respect. The wrinkles that write a lifetime into a face like a letter to the young are dismaying when one looks into a mirror. But this is the test, isn't it? How contemptuous I have been of women who try to look younger than they are! How beautiful an old face has been to me! So if I mind the wrinkles now it is because I have failed to ascend *inside* to what is happening *inside*—and that is a great adventure and challenge, perhaps the greatest in a lifetime— not sparing the rich or the famous, a part of accepting the human condition. At least, being well, I may be able to do better at it now than even a month ago.

Saturday, August 23

YESTERDAY a rather "too much" day. Anne Tremearne came late to photograph me because of the awful traffic, and I was nervous and on edge when she got here with a box of strawberries and lovely thin beans from her garden.

I need a publicity photo badly so I *hope* she did well with my old face.

I took her out to lunch and on the way she noted a wild

tall purple orchid by the roadside—Anne notices everything—later a large white egret in the salt marsh. I have only seen small ones.

After lunch she took me to the post office and the IGA. When I got home I found there was a slip saying an Express Mail was at the post office, so I started out early to pick it up before meeting Marilyn Mumford from Bucknell University and Karen Elias from upstate New York. I had a bottle of champagne for them in the fridge. It was a celebration of their meeting and becoming friends, partly through their both knowing me. I was one of Karen's adjuncts when she got her Ph.D. from Union College, and Marilyn I feel is an old friend too, since Bucknell gave me—*and* Carol Heilbrun—honorary degrees two years ago.

The express was not a letter but Eda's new book, *Oh, To Be 50 Again!*, which I opened to the dedication page and discovered that she has dedicated it to me and another friend. I am touched.

Karen, Marilyn and I had a splendid talk about everything under the sun. But after dinner at Dockside it was around nine and I felt awfully tired.

It is better *not* to have two social occasions in one day if possible. But of course August is *the* month when people pour in to Maine.

The weather has changed to a gritty wind, lowering sky—and I hope it may rain tonight. But I feel low and depressed—and only the animals are any comfort.

Sunday, August 24

IT DID RAIN and all feels fresh today—with a lovely European sky, big clouds with sun breaking through them—it occurs to me that this is not an effect we often see in Maine. There is often fog or a closed pewter-gray sky, or a clear blue one, but rarely the cumulous clouds, light-shot, which make me think of Suffolk and of Belgium where the sky is rarely still and clouds come and go all the time.

Eda LeShan speaks to the point in her book when she talks about the necessity to break habits that encrust themselves sometimes over the spring waters of a life. I think I must not allow myself to be imprisoned by my compulsive need to answer so many people—but the problem is old friends who are, many of them, far away, and keeping in touch with *them* is important. It is again my old problem of the immense number of beloved people who have entered my life for sixty years or so. I want to respond always, but the frenzied push-push-push has to go now. How does one break such an ingrained habit with so much guilt and pressure held in it?

Some years ago I went to Larry LeShan for four sessions as a patient to get his wise help about this. He tried to persuade me that I did not *have* to answer everyone, that the letters were answers to my books. It did help—but I fear I was not wholly convinced. My mind accepts the reality, my heart was warmed by his kindness, but somehow the spirit was *not* quite ready to give this compulsion up!

Monday, August 25

A BRILLIANT AUTUMNAL DAY with autumn's dark blue ocean and again some architectural clouds edged gold moving across the blue. The wind whistles around the house and I think of chrysanthemum plants and just called Edythe to see if she would have lunch with me and go and find some—although the traffic is bound to be bad.

I am immersed in Eda's book, full of anecdotes and the wonders and alarms of a first coming to terms with what old age will bring—for she was sixty-three when she wrote it, and it was like the touch of autumn I feel in the air today. Maybe that's when one can write best of autumn. Now I do not want to write about old age because I am there, I suppose. Yet I know that the challenge through a thicket of physical problems is to believe in ascension still and manage to throw the crutches away, so to speak, and the more helpless in some ways, the more of a triumph to keep carting away non-essential things and climbing towards death in naked joy.

Having uttered that I must admit that when I was ill I could not think about clothes at all, and now, yesterday, ordered a stunning purple suede jacket! But maybe the ascension can't do with crutches but does do with looking as well as possible.

The Nickleby reviews are splendid! I'm so glad for Pat Keen and the whole cast. The *Times* review ended:

For its entire duration, it enraptures the audience in a romantic, but throbbingly real world, moving us with an eloquent moral tale of the possibilities of redemption and regeneration.

Tuesday, August 26

SUCH AUTUMN IN THE AIR—it is exhilarating! Another "first" since my healing—I watered the terrace beds. I had dreaded it, dreaded being out of breath after moving the sprayer around, running upstairs to turn water off and on, etc., but I did it with ease. Before that I had done some more pruning and clipping. The garden is mine again. All spring and summer I did not even notice what was going on. I couldn't bear to have abandoned it. Karen worked hard and I wish she could see that at last the annuals are flowering—and the purple, pink and white phlox flooding the terrace beds with color.

Thursday, August 28

ON TUESDAY Edythe and I went on an expedition to get chrysanthemums at a place in Wells on Route 1—it was a glorious, sunny, windy day—and I felt quite drunk trying to choose three chrysanthemums—I was after spoon ones or daisies, the two kinds I like best. I did buy a Comanche blue flower which grows wild around here, a heavenly blue like a small daisy, three asters as they appear to have been decimated last winter. We had lunch nearby, lobster stew and strawberry shortcake, and then after going home and an hour's rest I went out determined to plant them. The earth was very hard in spite of my watering, so it was more of a job than I had imagined it would be, but I got it done so all were safely "in" when it rained hard yesterday. But I have a feeling the fibrillation is back—and it may be that I forced things a little.

When one has not been able to walk for months, taking life at a fast run is not a good idea—and that is what I have been doing! Oh dear—

Yesterday I got my flights set for October and November—and it all begins to feel real. Then I began to think about what poems to read on the theme of Ordeals and Rebirths which I shall be doing in Indianapolis and in Louisville. So the engine begins to hum.

Tamas, Pierrot and I had swordfish for supper—what an extravagance! But we all three agreed it was very good indeed—and for me the added pleasure of a glass of the Vouvray Pat Keen gave me.

Friday, August 29

BRAD DAZIEL CAME at five-thirty to talk over work on his essay on the letters to me he has been reading—a very perceptive job, but as he later admitted he had not really studied any of the material after *Faithful Are The Wounds*. I had hoped he would start with three fat folders labelled "Total Work" for in the last twenty years or more I get fewer and fewer letters about one book that has struck a reader, and more and more from women and men who have read them all. Brad has had a hard year for personal reasons and I think he bogged down about halfway through—and this is a pity because the most interesting letters *are* about the whole work. Maybe when things are better he will be able to go back.

He is the most loveable person imaginable—and combines that rare enthusiasm for the work of art with great percipience in judging and assessing it, *never* to display his own cleverness, I might add. I have the sense that critics write for critics these days—to be admired by each other—and rather look down on the creative artist who is rarely as clever as they are, but goes far deeper, Adrienne Rich, for example.

Later

I feel awfully exhausted, have cramps—the old merry-go-round or sad-go-round again? I hope it's only a passing "bad day."

Sunday, August 31

MY FATHER'S BIRTHDAY. He would be one hundred and one— hard to believe. Susan Sherman, so imaginative, sent me a little "Belgian" package with tisane, marzipan pigs *and* crystallized violets and a truly wonderful letter to help me cele-

brate the day. It is true, as she says, that I have celebrated
him and his values, but it was also true—and still is—that
there is a residue of bitterness at his lack of real understanding
when it came to my mother. Still, I look at his photograph in
my dressing room every day and am moved by that beautiful
sensitive yet wide mouth, by the sensitivity in the eyes and
by the great dome of a forehead. He was a whole man, "*en-
tier,*" not ambivalent, I think, and that is rare. The intellect
so fine-tuned and encyclopedic in knowledge, the heart so
innocent and unaware! It is we who were ambivalent about
him—so I see him whole and rejoice that I had such a father.

I slept very well last night till two—and then after three
for another three hours. I do think the fibrillation has stopped—
so I even dared get on a stool and reach up for the bird feeder
wire after filling both of them, then picked flowers, the snapdragons are magnificent these days, washed sheets and made
the bed up fresh, and now it is nearly ten so I must write out
the usual messages for Edythe and Nancy who will hold the
fort while I'm away.

It's a perfect summer day, and the sea so calm I missed
the sound of waves all night.

Harwich, Tuesday, September 2

WHAT AN ADVENTURE for me after nine months not away
overnight except to the hospitals to set out early and swing
out on Route 95 and then 128—the traffic low going south as
I had hoped it would be—and to come after three hours into
Rene Morgan's beneficent atmosphere again at Harwich. She

built this small delightful house when she retired at sixty-five, doing a bit of the work herself, and in these ten years, during her yearly stays from April to October, she has made it look as though it has always been here. Tall pines around it, a pond below, of which one catches a glimpse now and then.

How comforting to unpack in the guest room I know so well and then feel that I am allowed to let down, rest, obligated in no way. As a guest one often feels obligated, it seems to me, and it takes a genius of love to blow that all away. So right now I sit and write while Rene gets lunch. Perfect peace.

I hope I can put together the poems for my reading at Hermitage in Indianapolis October eleventh and in Louisville November twenty-second, "Ordeals and Rebirths"—perhaps epiphanies would be a better word.

It is an epiphany to be here—and I feel very relaxed and sleepy. I am rather glad it is a gray day.

Saturday, September 6

RENE IS THE MOST WONDERFUL FRIEND, cooking all the meals as though it was nothing at all—she is a little older than I but has been through two years of ordeal with Guillain-Barré syndrome. We went on little drives, one to Pleasant Bay, and Orleans, and the never-failing charm of the Cape touched me again.

At night it was almost too still, not a cricket to be heard, and I missed the breathing and rumble of the ocean.

When the house was built Rene had the oak trees cut down, so now there are only a few tall indigenous pitch pines with their Japanese look, but lots of bushes have grown up and her great success this year was a plot of wild flower mixed seeds, which make delightful tiny bunches.

I rested and rested, watched the news, read the papers, free of the mail which took me nearly three hours to read yesterday when I got home.

Sunday, September 7

DINNER AT DOCKSIDE yesterday with Mary Tozer, whom I have not seen for more than a year, and a Lutheran deaconess friend of hers who was delightful—such a peaceful time in the evening light. But I feel very tired and last night had again the dull pain in my heart which does not interest the cardiologists. My voice is somehow diminished now and I suppose I am in a panic about the poetry readings. For a time I really did feel a source of creative energy flowing back, but now everything I do feels immensely exhausting—even arranging two vases of flowers this morning.

In a recent card Jean Anderson sent me, Compton MacKenzie is quoted as saying, "the only mystery about the cat is why it ever decided to become a domestic animal." Hear, hear!

Shall I cut off dead heads in the garden this afternoon or come up here and struggle? By struggle I mean try to get the reading "Ordeals and Epiphanies" put together.

Monday, September 8

IN THE MIDDLE of the night, thinking about an intelligent but damning review of *The Magnificent Spinster* which has just come out in England, I thought out quite happily what I myself ask of a novel—the depth, complexity and reality of life *as it is lived on the page*. Not the "real life" but the author's vision of life which has been turned into art.

I have come to see that *The Magnificent Spinster* is a flawed novel, and not my best, though it is not a total failure. Of course the big hurdle was to write about Anne Thorp— Jane Reid in the novel—without probing in a way that could offend relatives and friends. [For that reason I decided that she must be seen from outside not from inside, and also that I would imagine as little as possible, and base everything, every episode in the novel on actuality, the actuality I learned through what she had herself told me or what I knew myself through our long years of friendship from the time I was her pupil in the seventh grade at Shady Hill School until she died in her eighties. But I created Cam and her friend, Cam to be the point of view from which the whole novel is told. Cam, not May Sarton, is thus the writer of the novel and this has confused some readers. The time came when I feared Cam was taking the novel over and it was then I made a decisive mistake to eliminate her as a character in the final part on the island, which should have been a kind of apotheosis of Jane Reid seen through Cam's eyes.

There is also, I am aware, a temporary dimming out when

Jane Reid goes to Germany after World War II. I simply did not know enough about it, and finally used a few of Anne Thorp's own letters from that period of her life.

The reviewers blame me for a "goody goody" character who is not believable. And they blame me because she is apparently asexual. But surely I did suggest that she could be passionately if not sexually involved. Reader, that is possible, notably with the character called Marian Chase. And selfless, loving and exuberant Anne Thorp was. I did not invent the goodness.

I am not sorry I wrote this novel, the last big novel I imagine I shall manage to write. It was very hard work indeed and twice I nearly gave it up. But I am rather detached from it now and look forward to trying a novel not based on a real person and to give my imagination free rein.]

There is too much on my plate these days and I feel rather shaky, but I did go out yesterday and cut dead heads, so that at least is done for the moment. It is very dry out there so I did a little watering, especially of the miniature roses inside the terrace wall which have done very well this year, unlike most things. Perhaps the wet June was what they needed.

Pierrot abandoned me last night and I missed him, but he arrived full of love at five and immediately lay on his back in the crook of my arm purring very loudly. That got me up at six, as I must try to do now every day, but even then time oozes away like water in sand. I changed the cat pan in my room, watered the plant window, had my breakfast with Tamas as usual, got dressed, made the bed and by then it was nearly eight.

I have nearly finished Jean Harris's book. At first I disliked something about it. She is persuasive about the trial itself, where witnesses perjured themselves, changed their evidence overnight, but somehow I felt she had chosen unwisely never to show feeling, to keep the cold, slightly superior "front" which the prosecuting attorney took full advantage of—and which must have entered the jury's decision: "guilty." The part about the Bedford jail and what jail is like is terrifying and very well done. The guards untrained and too young, some only eighteen, are insensitive and brutal, but so are many of the women. Harris's plea that something be done about the babies born to women in prison—some follow-up, some care be shown about them, is the most moving thing in the book. Here for once her compassion and true feeling as a woman with children is allowed through.

Wednesday, September 10

WHERE DID YESTERDAY GO? Mostly in going to banks to take money out of savings for the income taxes due on the fourteenth, then deposit it at Ocean National, then make out checks. All this induces panic in me, as all money matters do. With my father it was pure poison. At the very word money his face grew red! After that depletion of taxes paid, I called Norton to ask what the half-yearly royalties would be. Not quite as much as I hoped, but the first half, which included sales on *Spinster*, were more than I have ever received and certainly kept panic at bay during nine months of not earning.

In the afternoon I flung aside everything I *should* have done and went out into the glorious autumnal light and air. But the garden is bone dry so I first put a revolving hose on the terrace, and while it refreshed the right side I cut back the Japanese iris in their charming recess—it had been a fountain's basin—on the other side. Pierrot was fascinated by the arc of water being sprinkled about but only after a while rushed through to where I was. Then he looked darling with the long green swords of iris crossing his whiteness. He watched me with his intent blue eyes, only now and then put out a soft paw to play, but luckily did not attack as the shears were dangerous. Then, suddenly, he bolted across the lawn, such a white bundle of lightning speed, leaped over the wall, rushed back across the terrace, and that was that.

At just before six Pat Keen called to say that *Nicholas Nickleby* would close September twenty-eighth instead of November sixteenth. They were to have opened in Washington, after that in Philadelphia and perhaps Boston, so it is a blow. [For the actors it is a bitter end to an exhausting tour. Every actor in it plays more than one part except Nicholas who is on stage the whole time. The constant changing, often with no time to go back to a dressing room, and the perilous construction of the staging itself, innumerable stairs to go up and down made it a physically as well as mentally demanding show. The only good thing about this abrupt closing is that the cast may have been close to breakdown from sheer exhaustion.

I have always said that the theater is an angel with its feet tied to a bag of gold, and in New York the bag of gold gets heavier and heavier. It was poignant to read Frank Rich in the *New York Times* on the last night:

> As there are few more uncomfortable experiences, in life or the theater, than being asked for love by someone you don't love, so there are few sadder ones, again in either venue, than the abrupt end of a love affair that only just began. That was the particular melancholy lurking in the shadows of the premature closing performance of the Royal Shakespeare Company's latest "Nicholas Nickleby." Though this revival had opened on Broadway

to enthusiastic reviews, it expired a month before the scheduled end of its limited run.

Exactly why the show's producers had opened the marathon piece in the dog days of August—a time when no one wants to spend eight hours watching anything, let alone at $100 a ticket—is a mystery. That decision guaranteed failure by ensuring sparse houses during the make-or-break opening weeks. On the final Sunday, though, the theater was packed—in spite of the fact that, with typical haplessness, the closing coincided with Yom Kippur as well as with playoff games in both baseball leagues.

It was about 11:15 at night when the prevailing party atmosphere gave way to intimate farewells. When Newman Noggs, the beneficent alcoholic clerk, had his final reunion with Nicholas, he choked up on the line, "Nick, you don't know what I feel today." To which Michael Siberry, an incomparably openhearted Nicholas, replied almost inaudibly, "I think I do."

When the positively last "Nicholas Nickleby" ended, the audience pelted the stage with flowers. The company, disbanding after a year on the road, cried profusely.

If ever there was an audience eager to hug a cast, it was the one at the Broadhurst this late Sunday night. But the actors were to have their own private party. As the theatergoers filed out for home, a table laden with plastic champagne glasses appeared on the empty stage that only minutes earlier had been, as the stage-struck orphan Smike put it, "ablaze with light and finery." A more lonely looking table I've never seen.]

Thursday, September 11

YESTERDAY WAS a brilliant day but I never did get out to the garden. Once a year Polly Tompkins, who is writing the biography of the great South African white dissenter, Helen Joseph, and her friend Mollie Shannon come and take me out to lunch. I suggested we have a glass of champagne here first and a quiet talk, and then go to the York Harbor Inn, to sit on the enclosed porch looking out to sea. We have met once a year for five years at least. How I love these traditions! They give a long sweep to life somehow, an extended rhythm. Of course we talked about South Africa—and also about the problems of being a biographer—while Polly and I ate mussels Provençal and Mollie a seafood sandwich and a cup of soup. It all felt comfortable and fun.

But I had had to do the errands, get the mail, etc. before they came, so the morning fled away and I had about a half hour's rest and then made the *carbonnade Flamande* I have not made for months. When I came down from my rest I found a headless tiny baby rabbit and an agonized dead mouse which had been laid on Tamas's outdoor bed—an offering from Pierrot perhaps? I buried them under pine needles back of the garage where garden refuse piles up to make compost. It was hard and sad.

After I had the *carbonnade* simmering on the stove I went down cellar with garbage—Diane will get it tomorrow—and lo and behold, there was water on the cement floor. I finally found the source, which seemed to be a small tap over the

hot water heater, but it was too stiff for me to turn off. I called
Fabrizio and he promised to send someone. Two men came
today a little after I had taken Tamas to be washed. Meanwhile
Raymond had come chugging out to the field on his ancient
machine to cut the weeds. Mary-Leigh's machine is too big
to attack them as they are on a rocky knoll. I was awfully
happy to see him and asked him to come in after he was
through and turn the water off. He did it although the water
still dripped from the joint just above the tap. So, no hot
water till it's fixed. Finally when I went to bed the light in
my dressing room went out and it is too high for me to reach!

What did not get done was watering the terrace border
and I must do it this afternoon.

Life in the country seemed rather agitated yesterday!

I took Tamas down to the Blue Ribbon at eight this morning and brought the mail home. One very moving letter and
two *tomes*, pages and pages which I wonder whether I have
the energy to read. Royalties on the half year from Russell
and Volkening. Of the paperback novels *The Small Room*
seems to be doing best.

Friday, September 12

THE DISORDER AROUND ME is frightful—two big boxes of letters, two or three hundred that should be answered but never
will be, things piled up to be sorted out—a state of total
confusion and inadequacy on my part. Yet I live with it because the alternative might be worse, a compulsive "keeping

things in order" that would shut out life—and what is life now?

Yesterday I was watering the parched annuals—what a satisfaction! Then, the little border inside the terrace where white impatiens, lobelia and the miniature roses have done very well this year. Next to planting bulbs, I love watering— giving a plant a drink is surely one of life's best moments.

Life now is also lying in bed last night after a hot windy day, with the door open on the porch as well as one window— and air streaming through almost as though it were water, in constant cooling motion.

And life now is taking Tamas to be washed, feeding the ravenous Pierrot. It is writing to the few people I really want to write to—and shutting out the rest. So the disorder is all right, better than getting sunk and overwhelmed. These are good days because I am succeeding in quelling the compulsive responder in me. I say that and know that in a moment I shall be answering a twenty-page letter of self-revelation from a seventy-year-old woman whom I do not know. Ah yes, but the disorder is also the order, the natural order of making choices that are meaningful. So I can say that I'm a bad house- keeper but I think a good friend.

Saturday, September 13

POOR TAMAS FELL on his way upstairs for breakfast at six- thirty this morning and I had to half carry and half push him to the top which was scary. So I guess the days when we can

have that intimate time are numbered. It makes me awfully
sad.

But it is a glorious morning after two heavy rainstorms
yesterday—very much needed. Now the air feels washed, dry
and clear, and the ocean that dark autumnal blue. Perhaps I
can garden this afternoon.

I've been reading a charming bubble of a light novel,
Brooke Astor's *The Last Blossom on the Plum Tree.** The year
is 1928 and what delighted me especially was this paragraph
which brought back the Paris I knew a little later on.

> On deck they talked of many things: Mussolini, Maurice
> Chevalier's songs, Josephine Baker and Helen Morgan
> at their night clubs, of Irving Berlin and Cole Porter, of
> Henri de Montherlant's novels, of D'Annunzio and Mis-
> tinguett and Yvonne Printemps, the philosophy of Orage
> and the portraits of Bernard Boutet de Monvel, whether
> Lonsdale was better than Coward, of Gertrude Lawrence
> and Beatrice Lillie, and the magnificent Gladys Cooper.

What a lot of reverberations that list makes in my mind!

Sunday, September 14

EDYTHE CAME FOR LUNCH and we splurged by going to The
Whistling Oyster, perfect on this brilliant day as the scene
for a good talk but I was horrified by how undistinguished the

* Random House, 1986, pp. 20–21.

very expensive food was—even the croissants which were doughy, not flaky, and not really cooked. Only the dessert was good—ice cream on fudge cake with thick hot fudge sauce! Oh dear.

But I felt so queer and shaky all afternoon I got really anxious and called Edythe to ask her to give me a ring this morning. It seemed very lonely here with no one due to come till Nancy on Monday—and all this held in the image of Mary-Leigh and Beverly off to a cocktail party as I went out to do some gardening alone. Without the animals it would be too desolate. I am not and never have been a part of this community. There is no Unitarian church and even if there was I am not a churchgoer. I had somehow imagined when I came here, well-known as a writer—I was sixty then—that I would have occasionally been invited out. That has not happened. People come from *outside* the area to see me. The exceptions are Janice, Nancy, the Simon family who used to live down the road, and of course Susan and George Garrett who are now based in Charlottesville and are rarely here these days. Finally, as the Mercedes Benz went down the road, I went out into great emptiness and did some clipping of perennials— and that was the cure for a moment of dread and loneliness.

But the fact is I am always an outsider—we were in Cambridge; I was in Nelson; and now here. It has its advantages. Solitude is better than being bored, after all. I am never bored, only in some sort of existential pain now and then— and who is not?

Monday, September 15

CRAB MEAT SALAD all ready to go, and strawberries hulled, and I'm off to see Keats and Marguerite and bring lunch for the first time since before Christmas—such a festive day at last! Cloudy, but I don't care.

In spite of the two thousand amps sound that is supposed to terrify them, red squirrels are back in the house in the wall opposite my desk—and elsewhere. It is maddening.

Yesterday afternoon Tamas barked in his special "asking" way. It was not water or food or to go in or out, I discovered, but to go for a walk—and in the beautiful late afternoon light we walked slowly down to the sea, and I sat there on the edge of the cliff and drank in the marvelous deep blue, setting off the snow-white of the breakers—the coming and going of gulls. It has been so long since I have been able to do this, it was a great breath of life—and Tamas, too, rarely goes that far. Pierrot meanwhile got terrified halfway down and raced back to hide in the safe bushes on a small knoll. When we got near him on the way back he meowed his desperate "I'm lost" mew, but finally emerged like a thunderbolt and raced through the stubble of the new-cut field at about sixty miles per hour! I envied him. Then in the house he was totally exhausted and slept right through my supper.

The walk was a gift from life—how I enjoyed it!

Tuesday, September 16

IT WAS WONDERFUL to see Keats and Marguerite both looking remarkably well and the lunch was a great success. But I was too keyed up when I got back to rest. I had to read the mail and papers to quiet down, and then it was after four. I slept badly, waking from strange dreams. The medicine is in one of its harder stages when it affects the digestive system and I feel rather exhausted by it. Today I am very shaky indeed. A materialistic day as I went to get a skirt widened which I hope to wear on the afternoon readings—a soft gray and white plaid—it will go with several jackets. It's awfully long but that is the fashion this year.

There were loud downpours in the night.

Thursday, September 18

A SPLENDID CLEAR COOL DAY and I was happy, for my old friend Phil Palmer was coming at three for our yearly exchange of what has been happening to us. He had a heart attack last year which put him out of circulation for months and ended in his having to resign from a position he had hoped to be given and *had* been given a year before. Fate has been really cruel in this. Now he is back as pastor to a small church not far from Waterville. Luckily his wife can drive the twenty-five miles to her job in Augusta. He has been told by his doctor not to overdo but finds it impossible to relax. We talked a lot about what it does to be faced suddenly with extreme weakness, to lose one's *power*. He feels it is a gift from God, but I can feel this is a rationalization which he wants to believe but has not yet accepted.

I have been in the same state of "not being able"—and the frustration and depression it causes.

I was tired I think—at any rate I found I was stumbling over words in a strange way—substituting one word for another. That is surely an effect of the stroke.

What I envy Phil for is his seeing once a month three other pastors in fairly nearby Methodist churches—two are in their first ministries, one a young woman. Phil and the fourth member have been at it for years. For someone not married, like the young woman, the life of a pastor can be dreadfully lonely.

It's lovely to hear that Phil's son and daughter-in-law, who is also ordained, have six churches between them! Sunday must be an exhausting day.

I lay awake thinking about Phil and how he could learn to rest, instead of feeling he must read a book, or answer a letter when what he clearly needs is to lie down and let everything go for a half hour. It's interesting that I do not have that problem. I can sit for an hour in the *chaise longue* contemplating the changing light and relax completely. I have also discovered long ago that when I do that, it often becomes a fertile time when ideas for poems or novels pop into my head like those magic Japanese paper flowers in tight bundles which open in a glass of water. Perhaps it has something to do with stretching out on a *chaise* or bed?

When Phil left after an hour and a half, I was awfully

exhausted, but felt I must pick flowers as frost was predicted. Then when I was getting my supper the phone rang twice, and I called Lee Blair and Peg after supper. So I went to bed frazzled.

But there were the Yeats letters, the first volume is just out. These are the 1890's. None of his later arrogance is there and, much to my delight, he *hammers* at "clarity and simplicity" as what the good poem demands. With them and Pierrot, very affectionate, beside me, I gradually felt centered again.

The new heart drug is poisoning me just as the old one did and I have awful cramps day and night, but there is nothing to do but "bear and grin it," as my father said when he had a gall bladder attack in the middle of the night.

Sunday, September 21

ON FRIDAY I was really in great pain. It makes me so *cross* to find myself back in this syndrome. But it was a rather full day and I managed it somehow. At ten a publisher of Greek descent, Stathis Orphanos, who had written me a few weeks ago to ask if he could take some photographs, came with a Hungarian friend. I had dreaded it, and was afraid it would rain but there was a sort of pearly gray light which may have been better than full sunlight. Stathis is an enthusiast, and worked for an hour, his friend moving furniture around, with great concentration. I do need a new publicity photograph, although Anne Tremearne's are good and I was pleased with what she showed me. I felt very at home with these two men.

They had just come from photographing Richard Wilbur and William Kennedy, the novelist from Albany, and I was glad to know how handsome Dick still is at sixty or so. But as I watched Stathis and his friend walk down the grassy path to the sea, I realized that I felt at home with them in that special way because they are Europeans. What is the bond? A Hungarian, a Greek, a Belgian—what could be more different in landscape, culture, history, etc. I don't really know. It is some recognition of a common *soul*, perhaps—not definable anyway in rational terms.

Just after they left, Vicky Simon came. I have not seen her for months and could at last tell her what the pot of lavender freesias that I found in my room at the hospital after those six hours in limbo, had meant. She brought lunch, chicken salad, and a box of ginger cookies for Eleanor Blair whom she knew I would be seeing the next day—which was yesterday as I write this. When Vicky called I knew it was a little risky as I was bound to be overtired after the photographing, but then I think except for Janice and Nancy, she is one of my very few real friends in York—and I wanted to see her so I said come along—and we did have a good catching-up talk. The Simons are now in their own house, which her husband designed, and both children in school. Vicky works about twenty hours as a social worker with abused children. She spoke of how badly she needs her women friends, the three with whom she shared everything and who are still in Minnesota—an awful wrench to part from them. I understand this perfectly as my mother, too, felt in exile here in America since her intimate friendships were all in Belgium. Many women who have to uproot because of their husbands' job must feel this leaving of intimate friends as irrevocable.

In Minnesota years ago Vicky and her two friends spent a week end in a cabin in the woods reading May Sarton, exchanging the books with each other.

Her new discovery is Anne Tyler—and in that admiration I heartily agree.

Eleanor just called to say Vicky's ginger cookies were the best she had tasted since her mother's, "because they are real chewable cookies," not those elegant flat tea cookies people often bring.

All went well yesterday except for infernal traffic on Route 128. Eleanor, at ninety-two, looks rosy and says she feels better than she did last year although she has only now recovered from the broken left wrist a few months ago. Her house is always a delight to be in, the delight of being again with cherished things, with things that mean *a life*. She is elated—Lauriat's called while I was there to say her book on Wellesley for which she made remarkable photographs and wrote the text is a best seller—after twenty years!

But what I meant to write about is the garden. On Wednesday I let down after Phil's visit by cutting back perennials below the terrace. It was a serene afternoon, smelling of autumn, that particular tangy, slightly musty smell. It's crazy how much I have put into this garden, how little has done really well.

Monday, September 22

RIGHT NOW, however, the Japanese anemones are quite exquisite in a corner of the terrace so it was the right place for once. The things that have succeeded—let me look on the positive side—are five of the eight tree peonies I planted. The one in the lower terrace border is a marvelous pale gold with almost purple shadows and yellow stamens. It suffered last winter—bitterly cold and too little snow—but did offer a few marvelous flowers in June. A huge yellow pompon of a tree peony against the farther wall did well until this year, but the flower heads are too heavy so it never has the style and exquisite beauty of one of the single lemon-yellow ones at the back of the house. They are half in shade but have done well nonetheless. My favorite, a white single one, has not done well but produces one or two flowers like gods every year. So something *has* worked of all my attempts and failures.

The other success has been the de Rothschild azaleas, so tall and airy and brilliant, white, vermillion and pale yellow against the dark trees—one white one has a ravishing scent of cloves. The Japanese iris, too, has flourished.

But my attempts to get periwinkle to grow in front of the stone Phoenix and miniature cyclamen where the statue of Bramble now lies have failed.

Phlox did well this year, thank heavens! And the delphinium Raymond gave me for my birthday. The asters are out in the picking garden.

Wednesday, September 24

YESTERDAY WAS quite a day. First I managed to write a letter much on my mind, then at nine did a telephone interview for a Unitarian publication in Minnesota. I love the Unitarian creed: "In the spirit of Jesus, we unite for the worship of God and the service of man." I chose to go to the Unitarian Church in Cambridge when I was ten or eleven because Barbara

Runkle's family had a pew and I could go with her. We both adored the minister, Samuel McCord Crothers, a saintly white-haired man—we imagined he had a halo!—who preached marvelous sermons, full of quiet wisdom. One made a great impression on me—and really marked me for life. I can hear him saying, "Go into the inner chamber of your soul—and shut the door." The slight pause after "soul" did it. A revelation to the child who heard it and who never has forgotten it.

Michael Finley asked good questions, but I felt very tired at nine-thirty I must say—so much had to be compressed very fast and made clear.

Then at ten Nancy and I set forth in her car in a deluge of heavy rain and mist for Westbrook College to see the new library there where there is to be a Sarton Room, part of the Maine Women Writers Collection, which includes Sarah Orne Jewett, Millay and Bogan.

The library has been made from the old gymnasium and they were able to use some of the old beams. Even in the depressing downpour it looked most distinguished and exciting—the exterior a beautiful dark red with white trim. Inside it felt like heaven, so airy and spacious, I longed to sit right down in a carrel and be a student! The Sarton Room—what a thrill!—takes up one whole corner and looks out on a small white-pillared patio which will eventually be planted of course.

Dorothy Healy took us around, her eyes sparkling with pride. She has been the moving spirit of the college for many years—and it is she who has created the Maine Women Writers Collection. She showed us around, then Brad Daziel came and helped Nancy take the big box of autographed poetry books I am lending for the library opening—books which will go to the library after my death with my whole poetry library.

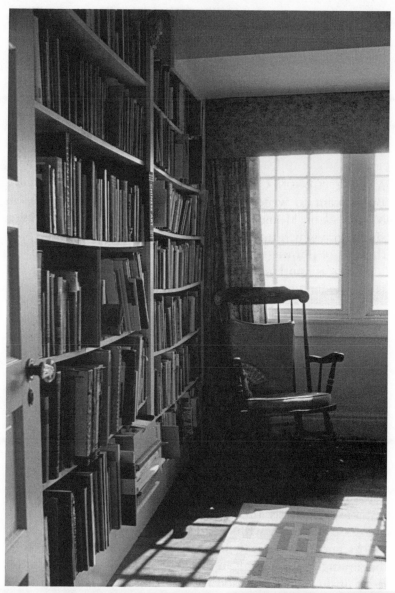

"my poetry library"

Thursday, September 25

AT LAST THE SUN! Calm glittering ocean—and my spirits rise. But I want to write to Juliette and send her an article in *Newsweek* on Memory which I found fascinating, including a single line which made me smile, "Snails hate turbulence"— the sort of phrase one can play around with for hours.

Here is another from Juliette's last letter: "But the truth is a very dangerous rock on which to put your writing desk."

Saturday, September 27

ON THURSDAY AFTERNOON I saw Dr. Petrovich and, thank goodness, my heart is not fibrillating as I feared it might be. The Westbrook day was exhausting and that explains why I felt so queer and dizzy on Wednesday.

Perhaps partly the relief of the good news did it, but I woke up yesterday with, at long last, the poem about the four ducks and two geese I pass every day on my way to town, beginning to form itself in my head, and in about two hours I got it down, and revised it yesterday, so it is *nearly* there on the page—a poem I have been contemplating for months. I jotted down what "came" in bed yesterday morning, and that makes me wonder whether I should not let that happen more often, lie there and see what comes to mind—before I get into the clutter and pressure of household, animals and finally my horrendous desk.

It's a real autumn day here, windy and cold, with a rough ocean that glitters like molten silver. When I came back from the doctor's on Thursday it was serene, so calm and beautiful, I went out and did an hour's cutting down of perennials in the garden. Perfect bliss. It is hard to describe how happy I am in the garden—the smell, the occasional monarch butterfly floating over the last phlox—Pierrot rushing in and out of where I am working like a frenzied *Comedia del Arte* actor— and Tamas coming to lie in his place under the maple tree. When I lift my head perhaps a sail appears on the ocean. Unfortunately, as I was trundling a wheelbarrow—full, to take to the compost—I saw Tamas and Pierrot standing together— at play? No. I was amazed to see that Tamas had a baby rabbit hanging from his mouth in just the same way—the animal, limp—Pierrot carries his prey. I managed to unlock Tamas' jaws and rescue the poor mauled baby rabbit—but it was going to die clearly, so I laid it on a shelf in the garage, the eye still so bright it *hurt*. Yesterday it was dead and I buried it under pine needles.

Tamas must have taken it from Pierrot, I think. One cannot be sentimental about the world of nature, but nevertheless, it is impossible to face such murder without acute misery.

Sunday, September 28

ONE OF THOSE DAYS when nothing gets done and time runs away under my feet—I'm not running but time is! It is very cold with streaks of sun through high clouds. At this very minute I must write a letter to Annie Caldwell in Saint-Paul-de-Vence. Hers is dated July ninth—hard to believe. The problem these days is not letters from strangers—there are four or five a day I often do not answer now—but letters from old friends whom I neglected while I was ill. These fine threads, the tapestry of friendship that goes on being woven every day, must be kept alive.

Tuesday, September 30

I WAKE UP HAPPY, longing to get at the day—and then energy gets frittered away taking rubbish down cellar, keeping things more or less in order here. That is a daily struggle.

Meanwhile every time I go out I am in a dream of wild asters these warm autumn days. They are a cloud of lavenders and whites and purples all along Godfrey's Cove Road—such a journey into delight.

Wednesday, October 1

WARM STICKY WEATHER—over eighty-six degrees here yesterday. I ordered my tickets months ago but when I went to
pick them up, found the agent had booked me to Indianapolis
October first instead of the tenth! She could not get me on a
plane for the tenth so I have to go a day early. But it may be
a good retreat to have a silent day to myself as I have been
invited to stay at the Carmelite monastery. I always feel at
home among nuns, and I look forward very much to this, and
am touched by the kind invitation.

Bulbs have come but I shall wait I think till late October
to put them in, so at least the chipmunks won't get at them
before the ground freezes.

Friday, October 3

I CAME BACK from my first professional sortie this morning.
A Book and Author Lunch at Darmouth College. It was foggy
but by the time I was out in the country the fog was only
making Chinese paintings with its swirls on distant hills, and
I came home drunk all over again with the beauty of this New
England. Everything I see now is seen freshly because I have

been away so little for nearly a year. But the soft yellows, oranges and sudden scarlet of swamp maples—the secret ponds and lakes hidden away in the hills, and the old gentle hills themselves—it made me homesick for New Hampshire.

It is a relief to have this first hurdle of public appearances behind me, although at first I felt like another attack by the gremlins that seem to be attending me lately, for I thought the dinner preceding the festivities was Thursday, and it turned out to have been Wednesday! Nardi Campion called on Wednesday evening as I was getting my supper—very relieved to find I was all right. Kind of her not to be cross, but I began to think I must be crazy—so it was a bad night, especially as Pierrot was nowhere to be found till after nine and I was stupidly anxious. He is so white he is really too obvious as prey—and the night before at four in the morning I had heard the awful shriek of a rabbit, no doubt being lifted away in the talons of the barred owl. Noel Perrin, at the dinner he gave last night, reassured me. He thinks an owl would not win against a large fierce cat.

What a joy it was to see Noel again! He has white hair now and writes often for the *Times* and elsewhere and won the National Book Award in the last few years. I find him an utterly charming man, shy and eloquent, beautiful in a subtle way. Humor flickers in his eyes. I have always, since we met at Breadloaf years and years ago, known that we were kindred. "We meet about every twelve years," he said. It is so fine to be at once so at ease as though we were old friends. He is twice-divorced and when I suggested as he walked me back to the hotel that there was much to be said for solitude, he said that his ideal marriage would be alternating weeks of solitude and family life—but it would be hard to make the transition back and forth.

He gave the dinner for me, Nardi Campion and her husband, and a silent young woman professor at Dartmouth who is a fan. I liked her straight look but she said nothing. Anyway it was an extravagant gesture for Noel. You have to be a millionaire to take five friends to a restaurant these days—and it was a truly festive meal at a French place called Une Fraise just down the street from the Hanover Inn. The desserts were especially marvelous, mine *crème anglaise* with some fragrant syrup of fruit poured over it, no doubt enhanced by a liqueur.

It was far better for me to be invited to dinner after the exhausting day than it would have been the night before—although I missed seeing Dick Eberhart and Betty and for that I'm sorry.

The day began at five when I stumbled out of bed in the dark in order to leave here and drive for two and a half hours to Hanover by half past nine. I made it in time to take part in a radio interview with Jane Brody—the health expert at the *New York Times.* Louise Erdrich got there as we were running out of time. I found myself on top of things and happy to be "at it" again. Brody is a truly committed person and that is always endearing. But Erdrich was the most delightful surprise, so quiet and witty, so generous—she talked about what the Hopkins Center had meant to her when she was a student at Dartmouth. She has five children and has already won every prize with *Love Medicine*—she is half Chippewa—and that was a stunning book but not quite a novel, rather a series of short stories strung together. What does that matter? Only I suppose that the organization of a novel is much more complex and harder to design. I liked L.E. tremendously and felt a thrill to be on the stage, for once, with two women I admire.

But I'm glad the Concord reading tomorrow is reading poems where I am able to create my own atmosphere and

Zeitgeist. They have had to move from the chapel at Concord Academy to a large auditorium, "requests from all over the East Coast," the librarian told me.

Saturday, October 4

A GRAY DAY HERE with just a streak of bright silver at the horizon where the sun has broken through. The air is gentle. The world feels very still and autumnal here. The animals are asleep somewhere in the house. I feel happy to have this day for myself.

Sunday, October 5

BUT IT DIDN'T TURN into a May day after all—a phone call at eight broke the morning meditation when I plan the day and as I water the plants, make my bed, etc., approach what I hope to do slowly. A phone call at that time shatters the creative person in me like a glass. Then the mail brought a request for a recommendation to the National Endowment. I believe Karen Elias is going to do something of great philosophical importance as she continues to probe the female psyche. I am happy to recommend her *but* it had to be done at once. I read it with the mail at noon when I was feeling very tired—and laid it aside till after a short nap. I felt once more that I can't handle my life. It is too much for me to be the crossroads—or whatever I am—for so many many people, never to be quite free to have my own life, to be always suspended on someone else's need. I managed to write something for the Endowment. But I felt upset, at cross-purposes.

Meanwhile I am reading Peter Hyun's fascinating autobiography, *Man Sei!* He has managed to compress an enormous amount of information into the tale of his childhood in Korea under the Japanese—and at the same time give a vivid picture of his droll, brave, sensuous nature—so we are entranced by being allowed in to this remarkable family, and into a part of history we don't know. But this necessity to read fast and write to Peter has also made me feel like a donkey being beaten, "Faster, faster!"

Peter was at the Civic Repertory when I was a student and director of students there in the thirties—and I saw him last summer briefly with his delightful wife and his daughter. He is such a beautiful old man.

Now in a few minutes I must set out for Concord to give my first poetry reading. Thank goodness the sun is out and I'll have a wonderful drive through the transparent golds and crimsons.

Monday, October 6

WHAT A JOY to be with Phyllis and Timmy Warren—Tim is Judy's nephew and they are really "family" for me now—in their old Victorian house in Concord, Massachusetts, only two things missing, Keith Warren, "Gramp," who is now in a nursing home, and the yellow cat who used to sit between Keith and me on the sofa. Keith, well over ninety, still writes wonderful short essays on whatever is on his mind although he is legally blind now. I slept in his room and felt warmed by all the family photographs on the wall, grandchildren now joining his beloved wife Barbara, Judy's sister, and their three children. Tim, white-haired and distinguished, has taken on one advisory job after another, an exemplary citizen of Concord, so I teased them about being "the Royals" of the town.

I had a short nap after lunch, got dressed, and off we went to the Concord Academy, a beautiful modern auditorium which looked almost full at two forty-five. I was touched and delighted to see Keats Whiting in the second row. She was ninety the other day and never goes out, but was driven over with others from Carleton Village by Anne Tremearne.

All of this felt cheerful and welcoming—Susan Sherman in the front row with a bunch of vivid red and white anemones for me—but I have to admit that I am very shaky still. It was not nerves but physical weakness I had to combat when I started off.

I think it was a good reading—though I entirely forgot to read the first poem, "Franz, A Goose"—and only remembered it in the middle of the night. I made a break halfway through and sat down for a minute, and that was a real help. It is so odd to feel and be so frail!

After the reading we all went over to the library for champagne and delicious pastries and *hors-d'oeuvres*. I never got a chance to eat because people were lined up in what seemed hundreds to get me to sign books. So many connected to me in some way—including a woman who had done the costumes for a production of *Trelawny of the 'Wells'* I directed years and years ago at the school—in 1940.

Jamey Hawkins and her friend sat beside me while I signed,

the dear things, all the way from Boston and Jamey not well. It was a kind of Sarton "Old Home Day" and I loved it, though after nearly an hour I felt rather bushed.

The good news is that I know now that I can manage a performance—so I'll leave for Indianapolis with more confidence.

I brought home with me a round basket of flowers and herbs like an eighteenth century bouquet, and the card read:

> Roses for Love
> Rosemary for Remembrance
> Mint for Eternal Refreshment
> Oregano for Substance
> Verbena for Delicacy of Feeling
> Santolina to ward off Evil
> Zinnias for Thoughts of Absent Friends

Tuesday, October 7

YESTERDAY there was a momentous event for me and that was to read Darlene Davis's M.A. thesis for Pennsylvania State at Harrisburg, "Johannes Vermeer and May Sarton: a Shared Aesthetic." I read it with amazement to find someone who has understood so well what I am after and has managed to relate it to the incomparable Vermeer in convincing ways. She used Vermeer's painting "A Woman Holding a Balance" as her chief anchor in the analysis and *A Reckoning*, my novel, as counterpart.

She defines the "shared aesthetic" as 1) light, so much the essence of Vermeer's magic and so often mentioned in my work; 2) the woman alone; 3) something that might be called the sacramentalization of ordinary life, the "ordinary" tasks of home-making. This work has given me great joy. Occasionally repetitious, she nevertheless uses a great deal of material, including *Mrs. Stevens Hears the Mermaids Singing*, and the poems with grace and wisdom. Now I must write and thank her.

Carmelite Monastery, Indianapolis, Thursday, October 9

[WHAT AN EXTRAORDINARY ADVENTURE this is and how lucky I am to have been invited to stay with the Carmelites! I am still in a state of blissful astonishment.

But I was rather nervous when Rusty Moe left me here. We had stood outside the medieval fortress before the formidable oak door for a few moments. When it slowly opened and a delightful woman said, "I'm Jean Alice. Welcome, May," I was unprepared for such easy grace. She looked like a college teacher in a blouse, sweater and skirt, and it never occurred to me that she was the prioress, as I soon learned. And when the door had closed behind Rusty Moe and the outside world, I felt I was in a happy dream.

Jean Alice put my luggage on a luggage cart and wheeled it herself, so we walked alone through the stone corridors and tiny recessed windows looking out on the garden or the cloister. We passed many closed doors which I presumed were doors to the sisters' rooms, and paused for a moment in the chapel, a simple chapel used every day, not the more formal large chapel I was to see later. My quarters proved to be the infirmary. There were flowers from the garden. I did not know it then but learned later that Jean Alice is the gardener and shares my passion for gardening and my madness in ordering seeds and plants when the catalogs come. But what I felt at once was someone acutely sensitive to the needs of others. She left me to unpack, mentioning that she would come and fetch me just before six to go down to supper.

The infirmary lets nature in as it faces French doors to a wide balcony and has windows on both sides, so I was with trees in a haven of beauty and peace. I unpacked and when that was done lay down, listened to the silence, and fell asleep almost at once. I slept for two hours and then worked a while before supper on rearranging the poems for my reading on Sunday. I heard a cardinal somewhere nearby, and saw a lovely big dog roaming around below. The monastery is enclosed in high walls but the planting is quite informal so it is rather like a park, at least what I could see from my windows. The sense of enclosure, of being separated from the world, is palpable.

Later I learned how privileged I was to be taken in to the inner sanctum, rarely opened to guests even during a retreat. Jean Alice had sent me a postcard before I came with a photograph of the monastery. On the back I read, "At its dedication in 1932 the cloister was closed forever to the public by Bishop Joseph Chartrand." Jean Alice had underlined "forever" and written beside it, "Times have changed!."

There was a reason for my warm welcome. Jean Alice had written, "A friend of mine who has read and appreciated your works for many years gave me *Journal of a Solitude* about ten years ago. You have been part of our stream of reading and reflection ever since." So I was being welcomed as a friend, with tender regard.]

Carmelite Monastery, Friday, October 10

[IT IS ALL SO SILENT and at first the corridors and many closed doors so mysterious and bewildering that I would have been lost without Jean Alice to show me the way down to the first floor where the large dining room is. There I was introduced to ten of the sixteen Carmelites and we sat round a big square table with a votive candle at each place. After grace had been said the conversation began and continued at a lively pace during the whole of supper. I was inundated with questions about my work and realized that some of the sisters had read a lot of Sarton. They were of all ages, each a strong individual. I did not dare ask too many questions but I did learn that they take turns, each cooking for a week at a time. That night we feasted on an eggplant soufflé, carrots and peas, and a light creamy dessert washed down with a choice of rosé or white wine. The atmosphere created by these remarkable women is both innocent and of great depth. How rarely am I asked such cogent questions! How rarely feel so at home, even to our sharing strong feelings about Reagan's policy in South America! About Nicaragua one sister said passionately, "*We* are the oppressors."

I was in bed by eight. It had been a rich day of experience for me, and I was thankful to be in such a haven because I

do still feel frail and a little anxious because of the perfor-
mances before me.]

This morning I worked hard at cutting *As We Are Now*
for the University of Indiana where I am to read it as one of
the Patten Foundation Lectures. [It was moving in this instance to follow in my father's footsteps, for he was a Patten
Foundation lecturer thirty-one years ago in 1954–55, when
he gave six lectures on men of science in the Renaissance that
were published as a book, *Six Wings*. He spent a month in
Bloomington. By comparison, my own effort is minimal, a
reading of *As We Are Now*, by request, and a reading of
poems. I am nervous because reading *As We Are Now* must
be a sustained dramatic performance and I quail before that
immense effort.] Probably I won't feel as ill when that ordeal
is over on Tuesday.

This morning I also planned the poetry reading for Hermitage here, got it all organized with the lavender slips marked
and titled at the proper pages, so this day has been very good,
peaceful and workful.

Then I left the medieval world and was taken out to lunch
by one of Anne Thorp's nieces, Helen Knowles Glancy, who
arrived full of charm and full of questions about *The Magnificent Spinster*, where her aunt appears as Jane Reid. I am so
happy that she liked the book and apparently spread it around
the family when it came out. She had brought a book of photos
of Greening's Island and of the whole family gathered there
for three days after Anne's death to divide things up and, I
presume, to decide what was to be done with the houses.
When I came back I was so filled with nostalgia for that vanished world I was close to tears.

Judy and I spent about ten days on the island every summer for seventeen years. In a way it gave me a feeling of being
sheltered, not responsible for life, what it does for me now
to be here in this marvelous monastery—where I am the

beneficiary of all the work the Carmelites do to keep the life here rooted in order and peace.

The chapel is very simple with chairs arranged informally as though in a living room—centered by a round table. Nothing showy—a great sense of intimacy with the Lord.

Here I am able to sit for hours just watching the light come and go. Today, a brilliant day, sun through the leaves which have not changed yet, so it is still very green.

Carmelite Monastery, Sunday, October 12

[IN A FEW MOMENTS I am going to Mass just across the hall from my room. Undoubtedly, it had been planned to place the infirmary adjoining the small chapel so the sick can participate. The liturgy on Sunday is ecumenical so a few men and women were finding their places and Jean Alice came over to me to say softly that I would be welcome to share in the Eucharist. I felt tears starting behind my eyes. It is the starving for true religious experience that brings on weeping. I cannot help it. I was rather nervous when I sat down in a corner alone, but was soon absorbed in this unusually open way of celebrating Mass. The priest sits in an ordinary chair and simply stands to deliver the homily. The hour was filled with joyful music: Leslie playing the bass viol in one corner, another member of the community a guitar and then Jean Alice's soprano soaring up over everyone else's voice. She is such a small woman that it is amazing to listen to her voice as pure and unselfconscious as a bird's. My friend Rusty Moe from Hermitage had been asked to read the lesson and there he stood in a bright red sweater and white shirt and that made me feel at home. The reading from the New Testament was the healing of the ten lepers, only one of whom, the Samaritan, the outsider, went back to thank Jesus and affirm his faith. And the homily was built around this story.

After the homily the priest sat down and, after a short silence, people in the congregation spoke as the spirit moved them and it felt very much then like a Quaker meeting. Several members had interesting comments to make but the most astounding was Jean Alice's gentle voice saying, "My hands are God's hands." The sentence reverberated among us in a long silence.

I had much to think about when I went back to my room for a rest and to prepare for the poetry reading at Hermitage in the afternoon, hoping I could do well as several of the Sisters were to be there.

While I lay down, looking out onto trees, I thought about what I had been experiencing here, and felt the powerful magnet a conventual life holds. But people like me who are given a taste of it cannot realize what such a life costs. These Carmelites earn their living by typesetting distinguished religious books. I was shown the big rooms where all this is done, the computers, the presses. That is one side of the work accomplished each day, but there is also the household to be maintained, meals to be cooked and washed up after, laundry to be done. The cooking is shared, but who polishes the endless polished floors, who waxes the furniture? Meanwhile, the true work of the monastery is prayer and meditation—that is what a Carmelite community is all about. I came to see that what looks so peaceful, so full of order, has to be won and rewon every day by hard work. I, as a guest, could feel the charisma because sixteen remarkable women had given it to me as an unearned gift.]

I must not forget to catch up on the last two evenings I

shared, first with Skip Sauvain at his home and last evening with Rusty Moe at his house. Rusty is responsible for bringing me here under the auspices of Hermitage, an ecumenical religious center where he is a therapist. I have known them for several years, first as fans, I suppose, then as friends.

Skip is a great gardener—as is his mother—how often this love is inherited! He has a small house with a garden at the back and an adorable *patapouf* of a dog, a delicious scramble of several breeds. Rusty's home is rather splendid, filled with color, high up, looking out on a river or creek through very tall trees. He had made a thick vegetable and meat stew which I'm afraid I insulted when he first told me, "I'm going home to make vegetable soup. Would it be all right for dinner with some bread?" It sounded like a few cabbage leaves and potatoes and I had come a long way!

But the open fire, and the good talk, and what turned out to be an excellent stew shamed me—and we laughed about my reaction to the idea of "mere" vegetable soup.

Bloomington, Monday, October 13

I AM A TOTAL FOOL—wanted to wear my white turtleneck sweater this afternoon and found I had left it at the monastery. I do want awfully to go back someday, so maybe leaving it says so plainly.

Rain again. When I was here at the university two years ago, there was such a deluge I thought nobody would show—but they did! A full house.

The reading yesterday went very well—a warm loving

audience, and a beautiful introduction by Rusty who read one of my mother's letters. Oh dear, it brought tears to my eyes—then the applause when I got to the podium was so welcoming, so long and enthusiastic, it was hard to receive without breaking down in this ridiculously frail state in which I find myself these days. My legs nearly folded under me but I did sit down for a minute and that helped.

Bloomington, Tuesday, October 14

IT WAS A HARD DAY YESTERDAY, hard to say good-by to the Carmelites—and then I figured out when I finally went to bed a little after eight last night, I had been with people for nearly five hours. First the drive with Harriet Clare to Bloomington, unfortunately in the rain, but it was open rural country all the way. Harriet has two bookstores, one here in Bloomington and one in Indianapolis, and had arranged the book signing for me. Her bookstore is called Dream and Sword (from a line of Amy Lowell's "Books are either dreams or swords"). She took me to her bookstore here before lunch and it was heaven to be in a feminist bookstore. She had Allende's huge novel which I wanted—and Margaret Atwood's just out book of short stories which they will send along. Such an open-armed, welcoming place, with a tiny room at the back where one can read or talk.

We had lunch with her manager here, Sid Razer, and a journalist and poet whom I had met before.

Then at four-thirty someone came to take me to a party for the newly launched "Women and the Arts." It was fun for me to meet some of the painters in it, one of whom is immersed in *Kinds of Love* at the moment. Her husband is getting his degree here in Comparative Literature. Mary Ellen Brown, who heads Women's Studies here, had just flown back yesterday from a Congress in Jugoslavia!

I had forgotten altogether what the academic atmosphere is like—and felt like a stranger. Tonight is my huge effort, the reading of *As We Are Now*. Susan Gubar is to introduce me.

We had a wonderful Chinese dinner—and a very cheerful easy time—lots of laughter. The dean of faculty, Anna Royce, made the fourth.

Laughing makes me remember that the best thing that happened on Sunday was to read poems to the Carmelite Sisters after supper with them. It was such a happy reading, fragrant with their intelligent warmth and love—and there was one hilarious moment when in the middle of my reading the elegy for poor old Scrabble, they all burst into gales of laughter and it was contagious. The line was

> Goodbye, dear Scrabble,
> You took much and gave little

But then when I read it again with what follows,

> And perhaps that is why
> You were greatly loved

they understood, of course. I loved the laughter although it took me aback for a second.

The *mal du départ* is over now and I enjoy being at Elyce Rotella's again with George, her housemate, her young nephew Mark, and their two cocker spaniels. Elyce looks wonderful—full of joy, plump, with curly dark hair—the most life-giving person I've ever met in the academic world—completely herself. She is an economist and has also been active in the

feminist group at the university, wears old pants and shirts
to teach in. She looks more like a student than a professor.
She and George are the kindest hosts imaginable—and my
room feels like a nest now. Always the transition from one
place to another makes me feel cold and lonely, but now I
have a photo of little Sarton with Tamas up on my bureau,
and all is well.

Bloomington, Wednesday, October 15

I DID A GOOD JOB last night and can now enjoy the last three
days here without such a load of anxiety on my back. The hall
was not full. Last time, in driving rain, it was SRO, but this
time we were competing with the Hispanic mayor of San
Antonio! I suppose there were two hundred fifty or three
hundred there. The audience was absolutely still while I read
in a good strong voice, thank goodness, and there was no
coughing at all. The hours I had spent condensing and cutting
As We Are Now really paid off—though I had to cut to the
bone and the balance between acute anguish and some respite
had to go. Susan Gubar gave a very feeling and well-planned
introduction. I do like and admire her so much and enjoyed
seeing her here for supper before the reading. Elyce is a
wonderful cook and gave us lasagna, and since she does all
she does with apparently the greatest ease, there is never any
tension.

Bloomington, Thursday, October 16

I HAVE BEEN STRUGGLING to choose the poems for the reading tonight on "Ordeals and Epiphanies"—it turned out not to be as easy as I thought!

Notes on things to remember:

The train's hoot and watching it go by at Le Petit Café— oh, so nostalgic!

The charm and excitement of talking yesterday at lunch with five writers in the graduate school. I have rarely conversed with such a rich assortment of talents—two have first books of poetry coming out.

The good questions a professor asked at the open discussion yesterday.

The sense of Bloomington as a town, the wide garden spaces, the beautiful trees, and the classic Courthouse Square.

Few people at the book signing at the Unitarian church yesterday, but that meant less pressure than usual, and I enjoyed it and having the chance to talk again with Laurel, the minister.

Then a delightful small dinner party.

Bloomington, Friday, October 17

AFTER ONE DAY OF RAIN, what luck to have fine autumn weather although the leaves have not yet turned—and it must be glorious in this tree-rich town and campus when they do.

The reading went well, an almost full house this time. I don't believe, however, that the selection of poems quite worked. It turned out to be more somber than I would have wished. But people applauded very warmly and stood at the end. I feel I have done two out of three readings very well, as well as I ever have, which is encouraging. I think I shall hazard California in April.

Yesterday a lunch was given by Marion Armstrong for some of the library staff and library school—again a charming house—but what delighted me most was to hear about her great-grandfather's farm which is still in the family, maintained by a group of nieces and nephews who none of them live there but share in keeping it up, and luckily all have different skills. What a dream!

I have also to mention the best dessert I've ever tasted, some kind of persimmon cake topped with ice cream. I had not realized that persimmons grew in Indiana—my father's favorite fruit. We always had one or two at Thanksgiving time in Cambridge—but they were expensive as they are still in Maine.

Sunday, October 19

HOME AGAIN to a blue ocean and the leaves at their most glorious—oh, how beautiful it is! But as usual I am beaten down at once by the avalanche of mail that waits for me after a mere eight or nine days away. I want time to think it all over, to savor a sailboat floating past, the evening shadows in long bars over the field today—don't remember that form before in other autumns.

It is the more striking because in Bloomington it was just beginning to change—though Elyce took me on a drive through real country the last afternoon and here and there the late light shone through orange and yellow—and was reflected in a still lake as in a dream.

Among the enormous mail I found a delightful letter from a stranger and cannot resist copying this part of it here. The town is in Kentucky and will remain anonymous.

This town was not quite ready for a single, female business executive. For example, after six weeks of labor in the yard, my next door neighbor came by:

N.   "I wanted to introduce myself and tell you that your husband has done a lovely job on the yard."
ME.   "Thank you."
N.   "You know, I don't see your husband around very much."
ME.   "Neither do I."

N.   "What exactly does your husband do?"
ME.   "I'm not married."
N. (gasping)   "Oh, you poor unfulfilled girl!" Even at my
               relatively young age, I am received as
               "damaged goods."

Wednesday, October 22

I DO NOT choose my life these days, it chooses me. I've been
home now for three days and these things have happened—
or been done: on Sunday I did a laundry, then came up here
to tackle the huge mail and try to sort out priorities; I began
to plan the spring tour which I now know I can do, so called
Rod Kessler at Salem College to say I could come in March,
and he called back yesterday and set a date; I called all the
friends, Lee Blair, Anne and Barbara, Maggie Vaughan. Then
there was a startling call from Roberta Scarabelli who is at the
University of Milan and who is doing her senior thesis on my
work. She had written ages ago to say she would be over here
in October but gave no definite date—and that call took me
completely by surprise. I had so much to do, was racing against
time, that I was quite angry—oh dear. She wanted to come
here "for just an hour" but that would have meant her taking
a bus to Portsmouth, my picking her up there, a half-hour
drive, and taking her back. I could see no such crack in my
already chaotic two days before Pat was to arrive.

Then, later, a call came from Connecticut about an interview for *Down East* which I have scheduled for Saturday,
November first, the day after I get back from Orono—mad!

Meanwhile on Monday Carol Boss, who is arranging the Albuquerque reading, called to say she is in Maine and could I see her and two friends. I had a hair appointment at eleven on Tuesday so suggested they pick me up there and I would take them to lunch. All this was yesterday with Pat arriving at three! At least it proves that I can get things done.

Yesterday morning I rearranged the flowers, gave them fresh water, and Foster's gave me twenty magnificent pale yellow striped-in-red parrot tulips—so I had a largesse of tulips and gave Nancy some to thank her for all her patient work filling out medical insurance forms for me. They are now bearing fruit with two sizeable checks in the last days.

The pile up is the usual one plus planning for Albuquerque and San Antonio and the spring tour, which is now in the works, plus Christmas as I get home finally only on December fourth!

I did manage real letters to Juliette, Pauline Prince and to Jean Alice, the prioress. Oh yes, also packed ten or twelve books for the Carmelites and sent them off. So there is a massive amount of detail to sort out every morning. When will I get to the poem about the Carmelite experience?

A perfect day—at six the sun rose, a huge *red* globe over a calm pale sea.

Thursday, October 23

YESTERDAY WAS A GOOD DAY for taking Pat to what must surely be one of the most beautiful rooms in the world, the New England Center's dining room, especially at this golden season. The building is set in a deep cleft, a ravine really, between towering cliffs, boulders left by the glacier, where all sorts of trees have taken root over the centuries. The windows are perhaps fifty feet high, set in octagonals, so one sits and can see a tree from its root up to its highest branch—the light on the topmost leaves, and far below striking a small beech tree.

It turned out to be Pat's fifty-fourth birthday—and I did not know it, but we celebrated with fine sweet and sour shrimp and baked Alaska! I have not tasted that and the thrill of ice cream baked under meringue for perhaps forty years.

We stopped off in Portsmouth on our way to get birdseed, kitty litter and paper-white narcissus bulbs. I have just arranged them in two bowls and they should flower when Edythe is here house-sitting at Thanksgiving.

There is a titmouse at the feeder—first one this year.

Weather incredibly gentle as the leaves begin to sift down, one thin gold disk after another.

Saturday, October 25

ON THURSDAY we took off for North Parsonsfield to see Anne and Barbara after picking up lobsters—a hazy, gentle day with clouds shot through with light, the kind that made us both murmur "Constable." It was a marvelous time, warm enough to sit out for a while and hear about the tame bluebird Anne had saved two years ago and who came every evening to be fed after he got well. Just before migrating they heard his "talking" in the maple and there he was, come to say good-by. It is astonishing, the faithfulness of this wild bluebird. He had five friends with him, but had not nested in one of the bluebird houses in the field, Anne thinks, because there was an ever-present hawk this summer.

Major, the large brown rabbit, is in a new, bigger cage and was sitting on top of his nest—a large cardboard box—chewing at it and not in the mood to be petted for once.

I had said when we arrived that we must take off for home by three—the animals were alone here, I had had no rest, and am trying to pace myself to stay well. But at two forty-five we had just finished the cake Pat had brought and Anne and Barbara were very anxious to take Pat down through the woods to see their two ponds, moose and deer tracks, and all the work they have done to clear it out down there. I said we had to leave. Barbara insisted very sweetly that it would only take a few minutes. I felt unbearably pressured and burst into tears and fled out to the car, beside myself.

Later Pat said a very insightful thing, "You get upset like that, angry and full of woe, when you have to say *NO.*" It was apt because I had done the same thing on the phone when I got back from Indiana and Roberta Scarabelli called and expected me to see her for an hour. She is writing a paper on *Faithful Are the Wounds* at the University of Milan. I had just two days to pull myself together before Pat's arrival and I simply could not do it. She had no car. Anyway I now understand myself better and that helps. Roberta called back and we had a long talk on the phone followed by a letter with ten questions I promised to answer. Relief that she called back, but now I have to give a lot more than an hour!

Tom Barnes sent me a very good essay on what I am all about by Dr. Kathryn North, a psychotherapist in Princeton, New Jersey: "Creative Solitude" (*Desert Call*; Spiritual Life Institute, Fall 1986). It was a great pleasure to read what North sees in my kind of solitude and why I am as I am.

Another happening has been a joint review of *The Magnificent Spinster* and Margaret Atwood's *The Handmaid's Tale*, titled "A Tale of Two Handmaids"—a review dealing with values chiefly—in the Fall 1986 *Kenyon Review*.

Tuesday, October 28

WITH PAT HERE—and it has been a seal on our friendship to see her here once again before her return to England—I am rarely able to get to my desk in the afternoon, which means that it is a scramble to get the mail in order the next morning.

But today, after hours of work every morning, I have at last completed the ten complex questions Roberta Scarabelli asked me about *Faithful Are the Wounds*. It was not the right time for this and today after a final hour's work I feel really spent. Nancy is typing it out now. Fortunately I found four pages of carbon copies of the letters I got at the time from many professors all over the place, including Mark Schorer. I had forgotten how generous the response was.

Only Harry Levin, sure that Goldberg was a portrait of him, poisoned the Harvard air so that *even now* it is clear that I shall never be invited to speak or read poems there! Actually I based Goldberg on a man I saw once at a meeting. It was hard to go back to that book and think about it after so many years. It came out in 1955—so, over thirty years ago!

One day Pat helped me plant a few bulbs and as it is warm and sunny I may put some in this afternoon after she goes.

It was great fun to work together in the garden, but for the last two days it has rained—in a way soothing days, after all the brilliance. Nostalgic autumn days—I enjoyed them.

Day after tomorrow the drive to Orono.

Saturday, November 1

THE TRIP TO ORONO turned out to be a wonderful time, the two four-hour drives there on Thursday and back on Friday were a great rest. I rejoiced and drank in fields and woods, happy to be away from the over-inhabited shore and into rural country where I even saw a herd of goats, as well as cows and many black-and-white steers. After two hours I was in "the country of the pointed firs" with all kinds of firs as well as the white pines that dominate the scene in York. The tall elegant firs pointing so high always move me. It was a clear, gold day—no wind—and the farther north I drove the fewer leaves remained. Most of us never realize anything about this huge inner Maine, the sense of space, and wilderness—of course interrupted by the huge mall at Bangor where I stopped and bought some Christmas wrappings. It all felt like a holiday.

Then it was lovely to step into Rob and Connie's house I know so well, its kitchen so inviting that guests gather there and look at the wood fire. Connie was not home yet so I tore myself away and had a nap upstairs. This time no speech ahead so I could relax and had a snooze.

The occasion at five in the magnificent new Arts Building, just opened, was the first Maryann Hartman Awards. It will be a yearly celebration of distinguished Maine women, I gather.

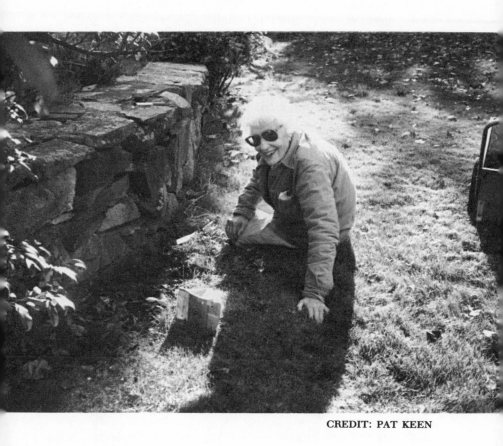

CREDIT: PAT KEEN

I was so happy to meet Berenice Abbott at last—also Catherine Cutler, a great worker in the vineyard of Family Services
and many other community services. Berenice is at once vis-
ibly a great person—from her enchanting purple soft clothing,
to the sturdy black moccasins to be seen below it—such a
keen, merry, intelligent awareness of everything in those blue
eyes under a thin cap of white hair. There we sat on the
platform, unable to talk, for what seemed a long hour. There
was a good audience, but the problem was the endless speeches
about first Maryann Hartman herself, then each of the award
receivers, with a rather long trio for cello, flute and piano, by
a nineteenth century woman composer, Louise Farrenc.

The three award women had to sit on hard straight chairs
being stared at all through it, and I found that trying to "act"
as a concentrated listener is quite wearing. But it was a good
idea to interrupt all the talking "about" people and have something really happen.

The pleasant surprise was that instead of the usual scroll,
we were each given a stunning gold pin in a little blue velvet
jewel box. Delicious.

Karen Saum was there, so we had a small talk and a hug
and she told me she has the old farmhouse she dreamed of
and has moved in.

Later

But the real celebration for me was supper "at home" with
Rob and Connie Hunting, a leisurely Scotch though we only
got in around seven. Then wonderful salmon, Rob's home-
made wine—and very good it is.

Rob has retired and seems happy and relaxed, starting his
day by walking over to the church next door accompanied by
his cat, Shah, a gray Persian with golden eyes, to wind the

church clock. On the way back they play a game of hide-and-seek. He and Connie together cut wood for the two wood-burning stoves—the kitchen one was lighted in my honor for the first time this year—so the garage not only houses two cars but a wall of firewood neatly stacked to the ceiling. The other day Rob was able to install a light for Connie to read by when she stretches out on the bench by the window, leaning against pillows embroidered with brilliant flowers. They reminded me of Colette's when she was crippled and managed to create such designs. But, no, someone she knew was going to throw them out and Connie rescued them.

Rob has also painted most of the inside of the house since I was last there.

All this New England talent for domestic invention delights me. Happy the man who at seventy-two—retired head of the Department of English at the university—can be at home with so many skills and, far from taking it easy, is as busy as a bee all day long like an eighteenth century "householder."

What will stay with me from this memorable trip north is Connie's face which I glimpsed in repose as the concert at the award ceremony was being played. Suddenly I saw the beauty of it, the clarity and something noble that her usual responsiveness and quickness does not reveal—a treasure.

I drove back in three and a half hours as I did not stop, took Edythe out for lunch to Piper's—which has replaced Spice of Life, now closed, as our refuge—had a nap and did manage to plant bulbs for an hour till four when the light fades these days. An hour of work is all I can manage, anyway, so it is just as well.

Tuesday, November 4

SINCE I GOT BACK FROM ORONO it has been on the wild side here. I did manage to get bulbs in, almost all the little ones, on Saturday afternoon after a three hour interview for *Down East*. David Phillips was leisurely and perceptive—and we shall see what comes out. It took three hours which I really didn't have, but I did work outdoors for an hour after my nap. It gets so dark by four I have to call Pierrot in—for after dark he disappears, becomes a tiger and won't come in for hours.

Janice, whom I have not seen for ages, came to have brunch—in her new silver Omni—a beaut of a car. As we turned out into the drive—it was raining hard—a young doe leaped over the orchard and away, a breathtaking moment. It is hunting season, so at dusk I hear the heavy ominous thud of guns—once, five shots in one burst. It makes me feel sick and afraid to the marrow of my bones. These days we are the killing fields again.

I can't understand why the gun lobby fights *even* for the Saturday night special—a gun designed to kill people not animals. It appears to be pure blood lust.

It is one of those times when gremlins are at work—mice in the stock of toilet paper on a high shelf tore it to shreds. Two light bulbs, one over my bed and one over my desk, burned out yesterday. This morning I fell with my breakfast tray—almost everything broken and an awful mess to clean up because I was having cream of wheat. The antique blue bowl that Edythe gave me is in smithereens.

But the worst is that Tamas is ill and won't eat. I took him to the vet yesterday. He may have liver trouble. But since he threw up last night after a single mouthful of cheese no larger than a fingernail, I now think there is an obstruction in his throat and am taking him back at ten-fifteen.

So another morning spent—I am terribly driven.

But it is Nancy's birthday as well as election day and we are having pizza here. What a comfort she is. I could never explain all that she manages to do for me from filling the bird feeders to extraordinary feats of finding things in the files. At least in her region all is in order, while here in my region all is chaos!

Albuquerque, Friday, November 7

HERE I AM, after forty years, back in New Mexico to give a reading tonight, and staying with Lou duFault and Rene Morgan—Rene spends her winters here. But there are shadows in spite of a brilliant blue sky.

Dr. Beekman called me yesterday morning at eight to say that Tamas had died during the night. Edythe was coming at nine-thirty to drive me to the airport. Luckily I was packed as I was in a state of shock. The plan had been to take him to the Angell Memorial in Boston for an operation to remove the bone stuck deep in the esophagus. Dr. Beekman had tried everything, even a scope he used with the help of an M.D.

I still cannot believe that Tamas has gone *forever*, woke up crying this morning, but I have to try to keep grief down or I shall be overwhelmed. I think it is best for Tamas—he had seemed terribly lame these last weeks, did not want to walk, and we all knew the time was coming when he would not enjoy what had been a wonderful dog life any more.

Something went out of the intimacy of our companionship when I was ill and no longer had the strength to cajole him upstairs at night. He was often incontinent as well, so he could no longer sleep on my bed, groaning little groans of pleasure when I turned over, and perfectly still all night.

At night I could be sure he did not have a tick and be in close touch with his physical being. I felt cut off in a queer way when he slept at the foot of the stairs, as he has done for months now.

But there was no doubt that his growing disability, his so evident suffering from old age, affected my own aging self. I thought of us as two very old people—but now that I am well again I am not any longer the very old woman with a very old dog I was all spring and summer. In one way therefore his absence is a release from sorrow and anxiety.

But oh how desolate the house felt in that hour after I heard the news! No Tamas lying under the table, his nose on his white paws, and those attentive dark eyes watching me.

I think of all his gentle ways—how once when a six-month-old baby was brought to the house he sat looking at it with pure adoration—I really felt I should give him a baby!—how when Jamie had a seizure and was lying on the floor near the flower window, held in her friend's arm, Tamas was terribly concerned and finally pushed his head under the arm to lick Jamie's face, and how she woke then.

Our walks through the woods when I first came to York, Tamas in the lead, his nose telling him a pheasant had passed

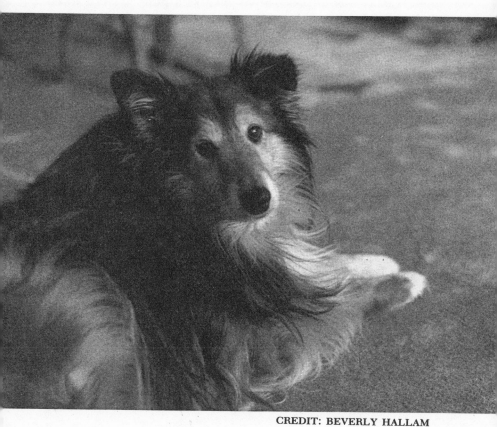

CREDIT: BEVERLY HALLAM

by—wild excitement and barking!—and Bramble following us at a discreet distance. We were a family of three, that is what is so hard. It is good that Pierrot is young and still with me.

Tamas was ultra-sensitive even as a puppy. He learned not to bark at Bramble, who had left the house when he came, and the day came when I saw him swallow a bark at the sight of her, and then we sat for a minute, Bramble on one side and Tamas on the other, and they became friends.

He was not a watchdog as he loved people—but let any dog enter his terrain and his tail shot up in an angry plume, his ruff seemed to swell and he growled and barked so fiercely that any marauding dog got the message and left.

His gentle spirit is no more—his death has torn a huge hole in the fabric of my life—my only dog. Some losses can't ever be wholly absorbed as I learned with the death of Bramble almost a year ago.

Last week I heard that Peggy Pond Church, the poet, had died. I wanted to see her once more, but she had written me in great depression for she was going blind, and for her it is best.

A few weeks ago she had sent me a last poignant poem:

> Now I, old willow tree from which the birds
> > have fled,
> through whose branches the sap no longer rises,
> leave my own vacancy on the waiting air.

Albuquerque, Saturday, November 8

THE RECEPTION by a big audience at the KiMo Theatre here last night was incredible. At first I had feared no one would come, in spite of the supportive group of women who had asked me and who were enthusiastic and sure there would be a good audience—and indeed there was! I felt like a sport star for when Carol Boss, my introducer, parted the curtain and I followed her on stage, there was such a roar, such prolonged applause, laughter, rejoicing, and finally all standing, that poor Carol had to wait quite a while to do her very fine introduction. I felt lifted up on a great merry wave of welcome and read as well as I ever have, I think—although when I took a short break halfway through, my knees barely supported me to the wing chair I had asked for. I can manage though. Two months ago last evening would have been quite impossible.

Earlier in the day Lou and Rene drove me around the neighborhood, with the huge, tough, rocky Sandia Mountain always in sight, half covered with snow, purplish savage rocks showing through. Merciless god; it is a cruel mountain.

Then we had lunch at the Marriott hotel with a glass of champagne and that was pure fun.

It is so fine for me to be part of this household for a little while, see Lou and Rene working together to make this house what must be one of the most hospitable in the world. One of Lou's sisters is the head of the Franciscan order and lives in Rome—one more of those liberal nuns who are changing the Catholic world. Because of her sister, Lou's house has been a haven for Sisters of many different orders, pouring through. How warmly my friend Amelie Starkey, a religious of the Sacred Heart of Mary, was welcomed for supper before my reading. She had flown in from Denver, working ten straight days to be able to leave.

Amelie is between jobs but hopes to get the funds to go on with her work with underprivileged children in Denver. As it is she can do it only once a week, but she is so full of fervor and conviction it is wonderful to see her again—wearing a tiny cross carved out of a soup bone by a prisoner in El Salvador—where she has been several times.

I forgot to say earlier that a young professor, Joel Jones, in the English department at the university, brought a copy of *Faithful Are the Wounds* for me to sign. He is happy because it is at last in paperback so he can teach it—feels it is a very important book. I was so delighted, delighted that he finds it relevant *now*, after thirty years.

Earlier this morning I called Carol Heilbrun to tell her about Tamas—and she reminded me that she had seen him when he was a small puppy and I took her up to the Frenches to see him with his adorable mother, a very small Sheltie like a fairy in her delicacy—and there she was with Tamas and three siblings. Then Carol remembered him at three months when I brought him home and set up a playpen by my desk so I could keep an eye on him. He was such a good puppy— he never made a mistake—and from the first night slept beside me, deliciously soft in his puppy fur.

I called Eleanor Blair, too, and was comforted to hear her voice.

Albuquerque, Tuesday, November 11

ON SUNDAY LOU AND RENE drove me through the familiar moonlike landscape to Santa Fe. I never believed I would see it again after more than forty years in which it has always been the land of poetry for me, "the leopard land" as I have called it because the brown skin of the land is spotted by juniper and piñon—and there they were, the gentle, magnificent Sangre de Cristos, capped in snow, under a brilliant blue sky. The air, the "crystal" air was the same.

Last night as I looked down on the sparkling city from the Asplund's adobe house, they shone as brilliant as Mars and Jupiter on each side of the moon, my friends of Santa Fe, almost all "gone into the world of light"—and I said their names like a litany before I went to sleep: Alice and Haniel Long—it was because he loved *The Single Hound* and wrote me about it that I went first to Santa Fe in 1940 and there he was always like a godfather to me; Marie Armengaud, the Baumanns, Dorothy Stewart—who taught me about this land and took me with Agnes Sims to my first Indian dance; Margareta Dietrich, Witter Bynner, Dorothy McKibbin, John Meem, Erna Ferguson and, of course, Peggy Pond Church, another star now in that heaven.

On the first afternoon the Asplunds drove me in the evening light to the Santuario, and there I wanted to light a candle especially for Judy—for Judy and I met in Santa Fe on my third visit there in 1945. We often visited the tiny church in the valley with its two towering cottonwoods.

So it was full of these memories and the joy of finding it still magic in spite of all the changes, when I met Agnes Sims again. Since she is a non-writer of letters we have not been in communication for years. And there she was, suffering after an operation for a painful back. I minded awfully for she had been such a splendor of purpose and skill in her art and of such intensity and authenticity in her whole being, always in her black Stetson hat, tall, striding along like a boyish angel. It was hard to see her crippled, but it was wonderful nonetheless to talk, and to feel like the brothers we have always been. Agi has three big dogs and would go home to curl up with them for an afternoon nap.

When I first came to Santa Fe—invited by Haniel Long— he arranged for me to be put up by Beryl and Ted Asplund in their small house on Canyon Road. It seemed, during the whole two days, wonderful to find them the same as ever, but now in a beautiful house with a huge living room full of flowers and books, and three delightful cats. I felt perfectly at ease as we evoked one mutual friend after another and remembered winter picnics and winter dances at the Pueblos.

Ted now has a small vineyard with a friend and makes fifteen to thirty gallons of wine every year. He has been a garage mechanic, a genius at it, but he is not the usual figure such an image might bring to mind, for he is a Francophile, a great reader, a man of passionate convictions, and of many skills. He himself built the guest wing where I was happily stowed during my stay. Beryl, now eighty, has been letting go of her many concerns: being on the board of the Women's League of Voters, the Nature Conservancy, and many organizations having to do with the preservation of old Santa Fe. So now there is more time to read, and to take to the road in their ancient comfortable Mercedes. We did so yesterday for a long morning in heaven, as we drove to Abiquiu and stared long at the great purple and red cliffs and wind-carved temples that look so much like Petra—the austere landscape that drew Georgia O'Keeffe here. She found "her" landscape, but it makes me wonder how many people there must be who never do—who have never found the place where work can be rooted and the soul come into its own.

Very surprising it was to come to the artificial lake beyond Abiquiu where we stopped to stretch our legs. Somehow water does not seem quite right—only the sky should be that brilliant dense blue, only the sky be reflected by shadows on the purple rocks, not on this gleaming surface, unnatural as it seems.

San Antonio, Wednesday, November 12

THE DAYS IN ALBUQUERQUE and Santa Fe were so heavenly, I can't complain of really awful weather here—freezing rain last night and fog. Dallas, where I changed planes, kept us circling for nearly an hour. But at last at around three we landed here and I was met with warmth and kindness by my old friend John Igo, from Breadloaf Writers' Conference days; Kathy Armstrong, Bertha Ann Pacheco, and Mary Cronin from San Antonio College. They had to be patient as did I for I was alerted in Albuquerque that my travel agent had torn out the ticket for Dallas to Boston on Saturday, and what was left was only a *cancelled* leaf. Here the American Airlines agent could not have been kinder, but it meant telephoning Portsmouth to try to get it straightened out, and finally I simply paid the one hundred eighteen dollars with my American Express card. So at last I settled in to the Gunter Hotel—vast, old—and in this weather, cold.

San Antonio, Saturday, November 15

THIS HAS NOT been as glamorous a time as Albuquerque and Santa Fe were, partly because the weather has been really bad. Heavy freezing rain on Wednesday kept the audience away and only about two hundred brave souls showed up to sit in the vast chilly auditorium. John Igo gave a charming introduction but even after that I found it hard to connect—a little dismayed by the lack of laughter from what seemed like miles away, the blurred faces of the frozen people.

The extreme cold continued on Thursday so it was out of the question to discover and enjoy what I longed to see, the famous river and all the restaurants and shops along it.

[I did not see the river but I did meet Jean Anderson who had flown in from Seattle to hear me read. I felt we were old friends although we have only corresponded, and during my illness she sent me beautiful restorative cards, more than one a week, and was very present during that hard time. Jean is a musician and conducts and trains choirs and groups who want to make music together. We drank many cups of tea while it rained outside and I was grateful for that unhurried exchange.]

Coleen Grissom, dean of Freshmen and professor of English at Trinity University, did take me for a short walk yesterday, so I finally saw the river and mightily enjoyed it though there was no sun.

Meanwhile Kathy Armstrong and her assistant, Bertha Ann, took me on drives to "see the town"—and out for two splendid lunches. Kathy and her husband recently adopted a baby, now two, and I loved hearing about that.

On Thursday and Friday I talked informally, first about writing a novel, then about journal-keeping, and the word had got around so the low-ceilinged, attractive room was packed and the atmosphere a lot easier to function in. There were even flowers on the table—and what a difference that made!

San Antonio College is a two-year college open to all high school graduates, and they are doing difficult but rewarding work with men and women who need help in the skills they will have to have to get jobs. John Igo, who has been recognized as a great teacher, spoke glowingly about his methods. While I was talking about the novel, one of his classes had been left with corrected papers of theirs to go over. John marks mistakes but asks them to discover for themselves what the mark implies and in this they help each other. I would like to be a fly on that wall!

Coleen Grissom had spread the word and was partly responsible for the crowd, I gather. As far as I know, there was no flyer and very little, if any, newspaper publicity.

Last night, after our walk along the river, she took me out to Trinity and the contrast was illuminating. Trinity is a beautiful campus alive with fountains, groves of live oak, a magnificent chapel designed as the hull of a ship. There is a Hepworth sculpture outdoors and also a Henry Moore. Here there is money and privilege, and the difference is tangible between Trinity and San Antonio College.

What a joy it was then to see Coleen's home and meet her two merry, super-active black miniature poodles—one of which climbed into my lap and licked my face. Coleen's cat kept her distance.

I had a short rest there before guests for dinner arrived, and we had a drink with a wood fire burning in the fireplace and then were taken out to an elegant French restaurant. Good talk and marvelous food made a splendid finale to this not altogether easy chapter in my journeyings.

Tuesday, November 18

IT TOOK ME from nine in the evening to one in the morning when I got back last Saturday simply to *read* the first class mail. It is like being at the center of a whirlpool after just ten days away! What makes it hard to handle is the diversity of what meets me here: requests to pay attention from dear women in nursing homes; from a friend going in today for major surgery; two birthdays requiring packages and notes to send off; a letter asking me to be on a Ph.D committee for Union College—hard to refuse; plus all the personal and business mail. Then, meeting all this, I must first look back with thanks for many kindnesses by my hosts and friends in Albuquerque, Santa Fe and San Antonio. So I spent most of Sunday packing up books to send and writing notes of thanks.

It is hard to feel so driven that I cannot even mourn Tamas although I got his ashes yesterday and held the surprisingly heavy box to my heart. I shall bury them close to Bramble's. Someone along the road handed me a newspaper clipping about the death of a dog. The writer quoted Lord Byron as follows:

Near this spot are deposited the remains of one who possessed beauty without vanity, strength without insolence, courage without ferocity, and all of the virtues of man, without his vices. This praise, which would be unmeaning flattery, if inscribed over human ashes, is but a just tribute to Botswain, a dog.

One of the letters I read when I got home was a letter from Amelie Starkey to Tamas. Here are portions of it:

We will miss you, gentle sentry. I see your picture by my bed and sadness takes its toll. Fifteen years of joy and faithfulness for you and May—dear welcomer, so unaware.

You came that Easter day with a limping run and joyful barks to greet me when I was halfway to the door. I stayed at least five minutes to relish the welcome and the joy *and* to calm my nerves.

I remember now, you, a loving brother to Bramble, aware of when she wanted to go in or out. I wondered as I watched May coax your limping body up the stairs. And I thought this—Tamas is putting himself through all that pain to comfort May—and comfort for those of us who came. You taught us well what welcome is. I bless you, gentle sentry, and I grieve, for you are gone.

Amelie is right that Tamas was a wonderful builder of bridges between a guest I had not met before and me. He eased the meeting.

Wednesday, November 19

QUITE A BIG SNOW, maybe six inches, fell in the night and
Pierrot is not amused! Bramble loved the snow, loved the
delightful clean place to dig a hole in, tail up, rushed up trees.
She and Tamas both played in it—Tamas half lying down and
pushing his nose through it sideways.

Snow lights up somber November. Nancy and I talked
about how somber it was here yesterday on our expedition to
buy a copier—which we succeeded in doing. Spending so
much money makes me feel drained but I think it's going to
be marvelous to make quick copies of anything we want to
keep.

Then we celebrated with lunch at Luka's, the friendly
Greek restaurant in Portsmouth—even to strawberry shortcake!

At the A&P I found a perfectly ripe persimmon and ate
it last night, thinking of my father who loved them. It reminded me of Proust's *madeleine*—the persimmon that brings
the whole lost world of Channing Place to life.

I'm going to try to get out to have my permanent but
nothing is plowed yet here on the estate so it's a risk—but
fun.

Louisville, Saturday, November 22

I DID GET OUT through the lovely silent woods and the trees in ermine cloaks—and so am properly coiffed. But that was Wednesday and for the next two days I concentrated on correspondence, hoping to leave this time not quite as haunted as usual by the undone. And I wrote seventy-five letters last week so things are not as awesomely "not done" as they were.

Yesterday I looked out at five and saw Venus, very brilliant and huge, in the early dawn, in the center of the sky over a shot-silk, bluish-gray ocean. A beautiful sunny day for leaving for my next adventure on the road.

I was astonished to find long lines at the airport—the Thanksgiving people already flocking home, lots of babies and tots—what a curious word "tot" is—and young men and women as laden with baggage as camels—a rather uncomfortably crowded plane.

I had to change in Dayton and looked down gratefully on the descent at the squares and wood lots of small farms—such a welcome sight. The white silos, white barns and houses make me hope this area may be spared foreclosings and disaster.

At Dayton the plane to Louisville was half-empty. I sat beside, one seat away from, a distinguished gentleman I had observed while we waited to embark. He was reading a thick white book I seemed to recognize—but what was it? I found out that it was QPBC's paperback of four of Sylvia Townsend Warner's novels! I told him how delighted I was and we began

to talk. It turned out that he has a brother crazy about reading
who lives in Northeast Harbor. He guessed who I was and
had read *At Seventy*—guessed when I said I was signing books
that afternoon. So he introduced himself, Cyrus McKinnon,
an editor of the *Courier-Journal*. Perfect weather as we landed
in Louisville added to my sense of elation.

Louisville, Monday, November 24

A NEW HAPPENING for me was to have the audience for "The
View From Here" moved to a larger auditorium after most
had been settled and waiting—what a procession of people of
all ages made their way down a flight to an auditorium seating
five hundred, and it was jammed. Then the young man who
carried a jug of water for me spilled it all over the podium
and the floor, and the charming English professor who introduced me—a woman—called for more paper towels and went
at wiping it up with such efficiency that the audience cheered—
altogether a happy expectant atmosphere when I got to my
feet.

I did do well. I felt launched on all the enthusiasm, extra
strength, gas in the motor—and did not feel tired enough to
sit down in the middle as I often do. But I cut the reading
down to forty-five minutes. It was after four-thirty when I
rose to my feet and there was more book signing to do then.

Saturday afternoon after just an hour to rest and unpack,
the book signing in the huge Hawley-Cooke bookstore was a
jam of people, many bringing six or seven books for me to
sign. I didn't stop for an hour and a half! Then off to a dinner

party arranged because Maggie Vaughan had come all the way from Hallowell, Maine, to hear me read, bringing two friends. Our hostess, Mrs. John Llewellyn, was just back from Paris. So it was a good example of Louisville hospitality to put on a dinner party that night.

I stayed with Mrs. James Smith with all the comforts possible in her charming town house, including an elevator, and on Sunday she invited a number of people for brunch, including some of the Hospice people who had initiated my coming to Louisville, although I was sponsored in the end by the university, the Council of the Arts and the Kentucky Foundation for Women.

But I wanted to go to Louisville chiefly to learn more about Hospice and to meet Vicki Runnion who had written more than a year ago to ask me if I would be available. She gave a potluck supper Sunday evening where all the guests were social workers or at Hospice, and I felt at home and happy to be with them—one of the best times I have had for quite a while.

Nashville, Wednesday, November 26

IT WAS A LONG DRIVE from Louisville yesterday in mist and at times heavy rain, but it did give Vicki and me a chance for a long good talk, as she had offered to drive me here. That and the whole day on Monday when Vicki took me to see Farmington, an exquisite house designed by Jefferson, where Keats Whiting's mother was born. It was then a plantation, but after the war they had to move to Louisville where Keats's mother married a Northerner, and so Keats was brought up in New England.

I felt the same rush of admiration and love for Jefferson's genius as we walked around as I did fifty years ago when I first saw Monticello and wrote:

> This legendary house, this dear enchanted tomb,
> Once so supremely lived in, and for life designed,
> Will none of moldy death nor give it room,
> Charged with the presence of a living mind.*

Down in the cellar where there were Christmas tree ornaments for sale, I bought five little white birds—for of course the fire last year destroyed all the ornaments Judy and I had collected. It seemed a gesture of hope and of recovering to think of a small tree this year, a tree Huldah is sending.

Vicki then drove me a long way through the gentle fields, punctuated by cedars, the many small farms which here at least appear to be flourishing, to the Mother house of the Sisters of Loretto. She had told me about Jeanne Dueber, one of the sisters, and the remarkable gallery of her sculpture we would find there, but I was not prepared for such original and powerful genius. Jeanne Dueber uses chiefly huge branches and roots of fallen trees—holly, sycamore, oak, even willow— which she scavenges and manages to lift somehow into her truck though she is not five feet tall. They are then seasoned for from two to eight years—there was a big pile on the porch of Rhodes Hall, the gallery. And finally she begins to find the heart of a trunk or root and works with it to create huge pieces, sometimes reminiscent of early works of Henry Moore. Jeanne seems to be wholly innocent of how to get financial help, was surprised when I advised her to ask for recommendations! I am determined to do something about this.

* "Monticello" from *Collected Poems*; Norton, 1974.

Jeanne Dueber is as compact and pared down as her work, and one senses at once that she knows what she is doing, that it has come out of years of very hard work and little support. At first the Sisters used to come and look at her huge pieces and shake their heads. She felt she had "made it" when at last a Sister looked and nodded.

Going there, finding this sensitive genius struggling and creating such marvels was a great adventure. But as I think over the three rich Louisville days, what seems the greatest blessing was to see Hospice there through the eyes of this remarkable young woman, Vicki Runnion.

She told me of an old woman she had visited for two years and for whom, as she lay dying in the hospital, Vicki sang all night—hymns, folk songs. Whenever she finished a song, the old woman opened her eyes and nodded, so Vicki sang on— until the old woman died in peace, companioned to the end.

Nashville, Thanksgiving Day, November 27

A THANKFUL DAY. I think over all the peak experiences of this autumn, starting with the spirit-nourishing days with the Carmelites. I think of being with Lou and Rene in their all-welcoming house in Albuquerque and Amelie Starkey from Denver coming for supper there before my reading. I think of seeing Beryl and Ted in Santa Fe and a chance at last to talk with Agi, of going to Santuario, so alive with memories of Judy and our days together in Santa Fe. I think of the kindness in Louisville, and the adventure of seeing the work of genius, the heavy roots brought alive by Sister Jeanne

Dueber, and of the wonderful talks with Vicki Runnion. And now I am thankful for this life-enhancing friendship with Howie and Mary Boorman, this serene house full of Chinese masterpieces in transparent jade, Peking glass—the great Kwannon who presides. Here I am taken care of as I am nowhere else, and it is precious to be allowed to be a childlike self who lays down every burden today, even to writing at length in this journal, and rests in "worlds of balm."

We go to Huldah's for the feast; she looked beautiful last night at the party here.

Nashville, Sunday, November 30

SOCIAL LIFE, however much fun it is, is not what one wants to talk about in a journal where gossip seems inappropriate. I have been coming to Nashville since Huldah's first invitation ten years ago—and in ten years one has to face the inescapable struggle and tragedies that have happened to people—and the elegant life-enhancing way they manage to survive. Here in Nashville, Martha Lindsey, over eighty, gives a luncheon party for a few of us tomorrow, for instance. At eighty shall I have the *joie de vivre* in me to do that? Grace and Carl Zibart have had their life mutilated by the death of their only son, but she gave a lunch for me, inviting John Halperin and Anne Street, where over Cajun oysters and rice we talked literature excitedly and all agreed that Anne Tyler is a genius. In York I see almost no one who reads, so this kind of talk is a real pleasure.

Mary Boorman has had many illnesses in the past two years. But here she is as luminous and life-giving as ever, like the extraordinary white Christmas cactus in her window which is a delicate snow-white cascade of flowers that take one's breath away.

Nashville, Monday, December 1

I AM HOMESICK for Pierrot and, really, for my own life again— for solitude. Yet I have loved being in this beautiful room with its peaceful gray-green walls with time to think about Tamas and to remember him as the extraordinarily sensitive being he was.

A young man who came to the book signing in Louisville gave me two books—Thomas Merton on solitude and Teilhard de Chardin's *Letters From a Traveller*. He wanted to share them with me and I have found Merton nourishing bread. For instance:

> To love solitude and to seek it does not mean constantly travelling from one geographical possibility to another. A man becomes a solitary at the moment when, no matter what may be his external surroundings, he is suddenly aware of his own inalienable solitude and sees that he will never be anything but solitary. From that moment, solitude is not potential—it is actual.*

* *Thoughts in Solitude*, by Thomas Merton. Image Bks., 1968.

I believe that my mother experienced this, recognized it, early in her marriage—and that I myself learned it from her. It comes up more than once in her letters. Curiously enough, once it has been admitted, one is no longer lonely.

In his preface Merton says:

> In actual fact, society depends for its existence on the inviolable personal solitude of its members. Society, to merit its name, must be made up not of numbers, or mechanical units, but of persons. To be a person implies responsibility and freedom, and both these imply a certain interior solitude, a sense of personal integrity, a sense of one's own reality and of one's ability to give himself to society—or to refuse that gift.
>
> When men are merely submerged in a mass of personal human beings pushed around by automatic forces, they lose their true humanity, their integrity, their ability to love, their capacity for self-determination. When society is made up of men who know no interior solitude it can no longer be held together by love: and consequently it is held together by a violent and abusive authority. But when men are violently deprived of the solitude and freedom which are their due, the society in which they live becomes putrid, it festers with servility, resentment and hate.

So, South Africa, Peru, Chile, etc.

Thursday, December 4

I GOT HOME at one in the morning yesterday—heroic Edythe having driven through a deluge to the airport, brought me home and then drove back to Boxford.

Pierrot was truly glad to see me and, while Edythe and I drank some milk and ate a brownie she had made, he sat on a chair at the table and never took his eyes off me. Then when I finally climbed the stairs to bed, he followed me up and lay on his back beside me purring for a long time before he went down to the end of the bed. Outside it sounded like a hurricane. Wind shook the walls, while rain battered the windows all night. It was so comforting to have Pierrot with me!

But as usual the enormity of what lies in wait for me when I have been away for ten days does depress and yesterday I felt like a mouse under a haystack. Among other things I had two recommendations to write for the Guggenheim Foundation. It took me most of an hour this morning. There are twenty or more dear people to thank for various kindnesses on the trip. I packed and mailed off eight books yesterday to some of them. A beautiful purple suede jacket I had ordered months ago came and proved much too big. Now that I have lost thirty-five pounds I do not intend to look like a purple elephant! But what a chore to repack and send it back.

I wonder when I shall resume playing records—it has seemed impossible. I fear the opening of that door so I allow myself to live in a clutter of the undone.

Today the sun was out—I never saw it in Nashville—but the wind is icy, wind chill below zero is my guess. Nevertheless Pierrot in his luxurious white fur suit was happy to go out.

Saturday, December 6

THE PROBLEM WITH MY DESK is the constant fragmentation—that my mind is a merry-go-round of disparate things I have to do and answer. One is to answer daily requests: "Where can I get a bound copy of *The Fur Person?*" "Do you think keeping a journal is selfish?"—this from a freshman writing on *The House By the Sea*. Planning Christmas. Wrapping presents. I did one for Catherine Claytor this morning.

Yesterday the charming living tree that Huldah sent arrived like a corpse in a long box. But it proved to be a perfect shape, and very much alive, and is now drinking water and seems quite frisky this morning. Also a beautiful wreath came from H.O.M.E.

The sun is shining, Venus very bright in the east when I get up at five in the dark and Pierrot darts out into the dawn, full of energy.

Sunday, December 7

THE *Times Literary Supplement* sometimes provides an essay that I can ponder for days. This is true of John Bayley's "An Involuntary Witness" in the November 21, 1986 issue—a review of Donald Davie's *Czeslaw Milosz and the Insufficiency of Lyric* and Henry Gifford's *Poetry in a Divided World.* The review concerns what the poet's responsibility is. Louise Bogan believed that the poet can't be "political." We had an argument about this in letters which I presume will be published eventually. I have been torn myself. Perhaps the political poem only succeeds when it comes from deep enough to go beyond rhetoric—the danger. I have been steeped in the personal. For the universal in poetry springs from the archetype within the ultrapersonal. I could not write about torture under the Nazis, for instance, until a cousin died as a result of Gestapo beatings—Jean Sarton. Finally I was able to write "The Tortured."

Bayley quotes Montale who said that "no writer in our time has been more isolated than Kafka, and yet "few have achieved communication as well as he did." Marina Tsvetaeva said the same thing more epigrammatically: "Art is an undertaking in common, performed by solitary people."

That is what struck me and what I have wanted to think about.

Later Bayley writes: "As with 'bearing witness', so with 'isolation'. Both are matters of result rather than intention. Emily Dickinson or Tsvetaeva—or Philip Larkin, come to that—are all examples of the solitary poet, and yet, as Gifford admirably shows about the first two in his chapter on 'Isolation and Community', they are also poets who create and symbolize the idea of a community, and with whom a community of some sort comes strongly to identify."

Later

When Tamas died I thought I had seen the end of disasters this year, but now Barbara's sculpture of Persophone rising from the ocean and its curling waves has been blown off the terrace wall and lies in awful shards and pieces on the other side—like some broken corpse. Could it have been done by a frightened deer come to eat branches of the yew to the right of it round the corner? I can't believe this has happened. The destruction of a work of art, new in my experience, is extremely painful I am discovering, for art outlives us—and so it is an attack on the future as well as the present to witness it.

Tuesday, December 9

I WAS SO STIRRED that I spent three hours writing a poem about the death of Persephone—"Death of the Work of Art"—yesterday morning.

Now it is raining, after snow and freezing rain when I woke up, a rather soothing afternoon. Perhaps it is a peaceful day because I steeped myself in the essay on Fra Angelico in this month's *Smithsonian*—it was a perfect opening to a day. The brilliance of his serenity which shines with such a special light through the blues, vermilions, fresh greens of his palette. I had not realized how marvelously he drew landscapes—Jerusalem in one painting.

Yesterday I played Mozart's Concerto in C Major while I wrote the poem.

Thursday, December 11

FOOLISHLY, NO DOUBT, I agreed to read the bound proof of a book by Stuart Miller called *Painted In Blood—Understanding Europeans* (Atheneum). I had plunged into Halperin's *The Life of Jane Austen* like a pig in clover—and now have had to lay that pleasure aside while I read this negative assessment—negative on the whole—which the European in me does not want to hear. But it is healthy to face the deterioration in manners, for instance, and try to understand the reasons for it. What I miss in the mixture of anecdotes and history is *style*—just that is partly what makes Halperin so engaging, but he is writing from admiration and love as well as knowledge, and there is some sharp edge of grievance and irritation in Miller's book.

It has been said before but hit me again with the truth that the only successful revolution in history is the American one. Maybe that is because we were so far away from our former ruler, Great Britain—and the British did not boil with rage for generations after it. I have been surprised at some French friends who wish for the *ancien régime* even now.

Friday, December 12

YESTERDAY I HEARD from Casyn Van Till that his mother, Hannie (Baronesse H.P.J. Van Till), had died and today I have been thinking of her and that she was one of the only heroes I have known. She came into my life because she read *Joanna and Ulysses* and was delighted by it. I still remember on a black winter day in Nelson the thrill it was to get a letter in a bold hand from a Dutch baronesse! Later she came to Belgium and we had a long romantic walk in the great beech forest, La Fôret de Soignes, and the next year I stayed with her for a week. Later she came to Nelson. Since then we have corresponded.

She was a friend of the old queen, Wilhelmina, with whom she went on painting trips—Hannie painted birds and flowers (she was a passionate bird watcher) in a direct, naturalistic style. A boyish figure with a loud laugh and an immense capacity for enjoyment, she was for years head of Queen Juliana's household, and her husband Hans, aide-de-camp to Prince Bernhard. But there was nothing stuffy or snobbish about her at all. And when I saw her last she was living alone—Hans had died, her two sons were married—in a tiny house in Eemnes, a small village. She had made a studio of a shed and there she worked, painting tiles and water colors of birds. One day her neighbor, an old poacher she told me, came in great excitement to say, "I must be crazy, but yesterday while I was smoking a pipe on the bench by the back door, I swear I saw the queen's dog run down to the river! Was I dreaming?"

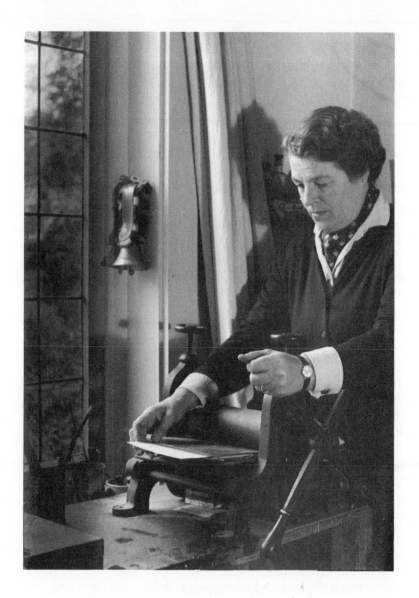

Hannie Van Till

Of course Juliana came to see Hannie, driving herself, and incognita—and Hannie did confess that he had not been dreaming. I can imagine the twinkle in her eye.

Why was she a hero? Because her husband, a naval officer, had been aide-de-camp of the governor of Java in World War II. Of course they were taken prisoners by the Japanese— Hans interned in a rather comfortable prison for men and Hannie in a concentration camp for ten thousand women and children. She was there for four years and somehow survived and brought her two boys, then four and six, I believe, through that hell.

Every morning in the steaming heat they were forced to stand at attention for the Japanese officers for one hour. Hannie often carried her sons on her shoulders. Those who fainted or died were never seen again.

Hannie's job was to make the coffins so she was taken to measure the dying every morning. How she managed to make them with almost no tools, no proper wood, nothing that might have made it easy, I do not know. The commandant also sent her out at night in a truck with soldiers to steal anything he might need—once, a garage door. So they had something of a relationship.

He himself went crazy whenever there was a full moon, danced and tipped over the huge cauldrons from which the inmates soup was dished out. So whenever the moon was full, a number of women and children died as one day without food in a state of near starvation killed them off. Hannie made the coffins but neither she nor any other prisoner had ever seen where the coffins went. When she managed to bring the commandant the door he had wanted, he asked her what she wanted as a reward and she answered "to go with a coffin to the cemetery."

He granted her request. It happened that the coffin that day contained the body of a child whom Hannie had heard feverishly begging for an orange. The child never got his orange; in fact, prisoners never saw fresh fruit. There, in the cemetery, however, a bowl of fruit was laid in the Japanese mores on top of the earth. Hannie, for once, lost her control, and screamed and shouted at the guards and tore the Japanese flag down. Of course she was taken at once to the commandant who struck her across the face and pushed her into a corner. She felt sure she would be shot.

Instead when they were alone he asked her to explain her rage—and she told him about the child and the oranges. The next day, a never-to-be-forgotten day, a train load of oranges was delivered to the camp.

Making coffins was not the only thing Hannie did—once a week she managed to crawl through the sewage pipes to the fence around the camp and there one of her former Chinese servants came to tell her the war news. Then she crawled back—through one mile or more of filth—and through a network she had set up conveyed the news to the prisoners.

She told me no one would have survived if they had known how long it would be before they were freed—four long years. And when at last the Japanese were beaten, a Dutch naval officer in immaculate whites flew in by helicopter, an unbelievable sight. Hannie was still wearing the one dress she had on when she was imprisoned.

All of this poured out in the times when we were together—and also the bitterness because when she finally got home and went to tell the old queen, Wilhelmina said, "Don't tell me. It is too horrible."

I know Hannie wanted me to tell her story and I wish I could have done it sooner—although perhaps she would not have wished to seem to criticize the queen whom she dearly loved. Yet she did tell me.

Heroism has been inherited. For she wrote me a few years ago, when her son Casyn was a naval officer on a destroyer in the Indian Ocean, that Queen Juliana had just called on the phone to say, "I have just awarded Casyn the highest decoration in my power for his heroic saving, at the risk of his life, of a man who had jumped overboard."

It is hard to believe that Hannie is dead—so vital, so alive she was—although the last years have been hard, her legs paralyzed from diabetes. May you rest in peace, H.P.J. Baronnesse van Till-Tutein Nolthenius, and may there be lots of birds you have never seen on earth, in heaven!

Saturday, December 13

I TREASURE what my old friend Patience Ross wrote in a Christmas message from England. Now in her eighties, she was my agent in London from 1939 on, until she retired.

> I know it's useless to bid you save your energies—and in a way, making the effort generates the needed strength—as I hope it will be for me. You have always been a giver—a source-person—making time (one's only unstorable wealth) for so many, yet always as one-to-one with your whole self. I want to thank you so much for that unique gift—and to honour you for your great Act of Work in your whole life.

Could I ever receive a better Christmas present than that?

Wednesday, December 17

QUITE A FALL OF SNOW— Pierrot dashed out into it and was gone for an hour, then spent a long time licking his big paws.

It's hard to write here when my desk is so crowded with lists of "not to forget"—but one of the best things about Christmas is hearing from friends like Liz Knies in Japan.

On Monday I had a lovely adventure. I'm so rarely out at night that I was dazzled, as I drove into Portsmouth to have dinner with Dorothy Molnar, little Sarton's mother, by all the lights and lit-up trees all over York. I felt like a child at a feast of lights. The most beautiful are the white clapboard houses where the decoration is a single candle in each window. I came home via Kittery and there too are prodigies of invention. The poorest houses have become magic palaces, sometimes windows and doors outlined in many colored lights. Sometimes a single tree has been decorated with tiny white lights.

It reminded me that Judy and I in the old Cambridge days always went out on Christmas Eve for a walk across Massachusetts Avenue where people were not academics and the houses were all lit up.

Later

I saw Dr. Petrovich at noon, the first visit since August and
he was surprised and happy to find my heart beating away in
sync. So to celebrate this excellent report I have made brownies to take to Eleanor Blair if we don't have the big storm
which is expected. It's very white and black outside now, dark
clouds over a dark gray ocean, and new snow, about two
inches, that fell last night.

Bill Heyen has sent a wonderful Christmas poem—the
first time I have felt that shiver in my bones of what Christmas
is all about:

Lord
of poised rocks shimmering in moonshine,
Lord of matter, and more,
Lord of being,
Lord of myself and the deep notes of tides,
creatures, trees tending toward me
almost beyond hearing,
reciprocal Lord of nothing, and all,
Lord of mica,
Lord of the harbor's light and haze,
I place this song
in my trembling book of praise.

Thursday, December 18

ONE OF THOSE DAYS when gremlins are hard at work! The refrigerator is not defrosting. I'm waiting for a man to come, and actually found someone who says he will; the roof of the closed-in porch where I live when I am not up here in my study leaks—so three containers now are strewn around, nothing to do till the ice melts, I guess. Bruce Woods, the nicest man in the world, has been here to put in two extra plugs in the attic, so the sound machine that terrifies red squirrels can be plugged in there and the wire not go under the door to the office—and getting a plug to work in the office so I can get Nancy some proper light. Eleanor is here cleaning!

It is now ten in the morning and I'm exhausted, but Nancy and I did manage to set up the adorable small tree in the library and the wreath hung, so that room is on the way to Christmas. Pierrot meanwhile has had a fine morning rushing about up and down stairs and into everything.

The expected storm makes me rather nervous about the trip to Cambridge this afternoon and then Wellesley tomorrow from there—and I slept badly, wondering whether to call it off.

Sunday, December 21

NOW IT IS SUNDAY—the porch roof is still leaking but is gradually drying out, but the fridge is working again and a new fan will be installed before noon. Again such a comforting man came to work on it. So things are more or less under control.

The storm was rain not snow. Had it been snow about twenty-two inches would have piled in! But the driving rain from the southeast made the leak worse and Edythe had to bring in a tall rubbish can from the kitchen. In Cambridge in the familiar guest room at Cora DuBois's, I listened to the rain lashing the windows and wondered what was happening here.

It was an interesting contrast to be first with Cora and Jeanne Taylor and then to drive off to have lunch with Eleanor Blair in Wellesley on Friday. Cora is now eighty-five and Jeanne my age, and Jeanne has to do everything now, even to cooking dinner, although Cora lays things out, peels potatoes, etc., ahead of time. Cora suffers from a rather despairing old age, is glum, and with some reason as her good eye was operated on unsuccessfully some years ago. As a famous anthropologist, to be deprived of reading for more than an hour or so is frustrating, to put it mildly. She had major intestinal surgery for cancer two years ago. "I am a recluse," she says, and it is true for she stays at home all the time. How does Jeanne survive? I admire her spirit for she is determined not to sink into lethargy, the quagmire, and manages to do some writing, to go out, to see friends.

But who really lives in that house now? Only the adored tiger cat who is suddenly thin—I have not been there for a year of course—and old though his luminous eyes do not waver. But it is tragic to see Cora so wasted—having in some deep way repudiated her own life.

It was walking right into life to walk into Eleanor Blair's little house in Wellesley and to be warmly welcomed—and there was such a Christmasy feeling everywhere I looked: a tiny tree in the front parlor, already decorated and with presents around it. Eleanor's eyes were shining and we had a good talk over our sherry, but Mitzi, her cat, was nowhere to be seen and did not come up from the cellar while I was there. Eleanor still manages alone but what she needs is someone who will read aloud to her. For instance, mail piles up and sometimes it is days before anyone turns up. A regular visitor to do a few odd jobs would do the trick.

She is still delighted by, for instance, her geranium window where Mitzi loves to sit. She listens to "All Things Considered" and also to the books for the blind which are read aloud. She is very aware politically and in fact is alive in the sense of enjoying life. She will be ninety-three next summer.

Monday, December 22

I NEVER DID FINISH because Jabber called from St. Louis and Karen Hodges in Texas returned my call. Karen and I have been out of touch for over a year, so I was relieved to hear that things go well with her and that Emily is applying to several colleges in the East, including Wellesley where Karen graduated with honors. Christmas does bring in the network scattered all over the country. After supper Doris called from Berkeley.

But the best event of the day was at eleven in the morning when Edythe came for our yearly decorating of the tree, this year a small elegant tree with a perfect cone shape. The image of last year's tree burning up is in everyone's mind. I discovered that far from all the ornaments being destroyed, there are still quite a few left. How did they survive? For a second, looking at boxes filled with the shiny ornaments—red, gold, blue, green—which used to be so common and are now unobtainable, I felt under a spell as though they had been re-created by some magic wand—the loaves and the fishes. I thought there was nothing left to save. The tree went up in a few seconds—filling the room with terrifying black smoke. How did I manage to put it out? Thanks partly to Mary-Leigh's placing of large fire extinguishers on each floor. Partly to my wild fear that the whole house might go.

Anyway, yesterday Edythe and I had fun savoring the tiny ornaments I had bought in Louisville and elsewhere. This exquisite tree is not easy to deck because it has been shaped and thick needles rather than supportive twigs and branches are slippery for hanging on ornaments. Many we simply laid on the tree, a mouse in a sleeping bag for one. I was happy to find the reindeer in a glass bauble safe and sound and especially, *mirabile dictu*, the star Judy and I always had on our tree.

I had written ten or twelve notes that morning before eleven and was tired—by afternoon a deflated wreck. I rested for two hours. A rough night as I had a hacking cough which has turned into a real head cold today, and poor Pierrot threw up lavishly on three rugs in the middle of the night.

Wednesday, December 24

I FEEL RATHER STARVED for time and space, although the sun is out and the fuchsia is out, today, against hard weather. How to try to keep afloat and not simply drown in the wild accumulations that Christmas brings to this house? Little by little, it fills up with chocolates, presents for under the tree, long letters and innumerable cards, and while it does I feel poorer all the time—and rich only in lists of what still has to be done. Chiefly more white candles if I can find them, oysters for Lee tonight—scalloped oysters were Judy's and my usual Christmas Eve fare for supper—a chicken to roast for tomorrow, and the tenderloin roast for the twenty-sixth when Anne and Barbara come. I dashed into Portsmouth and got vegetables yesterday—and hoped for persimmons but there were none.

In a way having my hair done is good—I *have* to sit down for a half hour there and glance through the mail. Two days ago it took me two hours to read it and it was too much for me. By half past one my old bones only long for rest. And perhaps also for one central person instead of this multitude— why? Because my response can't be in depth, and the cards I send out are hardly more than a word to say I am well again. Guilt and starvation move in.

Last year a fan made cards, and sent me a few. The message was a quote from somewhere in the journals: "Everyone at a certain point in the pre-Christmas shuffle must long to

. . . think quietly about friends and loves and ways toward renewal. . . ."

It made me feel better to copy it out.

And now to answer . . . one or two of the multitude.

Saturday, December 27

LEE LEFT EARLY this morning. It was awfully good to see her after a whole year—for I was too ill to have her here on my birthday—but I have laryngitis, have warded off a bad cold with aspirin, but the three days of Christmas here were a little too much. I kept feeling I was being buried under paper, wrapping, *things, food.* Two big dinners to cook on the *day* for Janice, Edythe, Lee and me and then yesterday for Lee, Janice, Anne and Barbara. The table looked beautiful with a white cloth strewn with violets—the pattern is violets—two deep red roses in the center with the silver candlesticks and tall white candles. The tenderloin roast about which I felt terribly anxious turned out perfectly. We had a great Haut-Médoc Bordeaux Lee had brought, and for dessert vanilla ice cream with *crème de menthe* and pineapple macadamia cake from Joan Palevsky.

Why do I talk about food when it was the spiritual food of being together and the good talk that really nourished? Why I talk about it is that I realize the energy expended reduces even my spiritual hunger to near zero.

So the magic moment came last night when I was turning out lights alone downstairs and for a moment stood in the library with only the small tree lit up, a poignant light—very beautiful and quieting. Alone with the tree I felt suddenly at peace.

I have just answered a letter from Jean Anderson in Se-attle—she who sent me a fabulous huge box filled with red and white packages of Belgian goodies, and even a card of Ghent. It took my breath away when I opened it. I really am a spoiled old critter.

But even more of a present was this she sent me by Rene Daumel:

> You cannot stay on the summit forever,
>   you just have to come down again.
> So why bother in the first place?
> There is an art of conducting oneself
>   in the
> lower regime by the memory of what we
>   saw higher up.
> When one can no longer see, we can
>   at least still know.

Sunday, December 28

YESTERDAY I WAS A FAILURE and was swept by a storm of tears, facing what is on this desk, what must be answered, what will never be answered although it should be. I have lived now for more than a month in a sort of dry frustration. I feel unable to deal with my life, with the too-muchness of it. All through December I have gone to bed with books in proof I am asked to blurb, first the one about Europe that made me feel so ambivalent and cross, now for the last week

Mary Elsie Robertson's novel *Family Life*. This is a very good novel and will be easy to praise but I felt imprisoned, shackled when I went to bed exhausted and could not choose what to read—Elizabeth Bowen's collected essays, two novels by Primo Levi I long to get at.

When Mary DeShazer's book *Inspiring Women* arrived a few days ago, I was exhilarated to see it out (Pergamon Press). It is about the muse as Bogan, H.D., Sarton, Rich and Lorde have experienced her. Of course I read the chapter on me first—no time yet to read it all as I shall of course. It is a fascinating book. Then when I read the later chapter on my friendship with Bogan, it was like a drop of poison and gave me sleepless nights. It is time perhaps that the question was asked, "Why did Bogan never give Sarton credit for her work? Why is the tone patronizing?"

During the time we were friends my book of poems *In Time Like Air* was a candidate for the National Book Award and in the same year my novel *Faithful Are the Wounds* was a candidate. I know of no other writer who had two books in two genres nominated in the same year.

It has taken me a long time to be honest about Louise Bogan because I loved and admired her so much. But now at nearly seventy-five I must admit that the explanation may well be jealousy. At a time when she almost ceased to write poems, I was producing a lot, in three fields. Chapters of *I Knew a Phoenix* were appearing in *The New Yorker* the year after I began seeing her.

I am tired of everyone—under Limmer's delighted guidance—quoting a letter Bogan wrote to Limmer that said "If only she [Sarton] would stop writing sentimental poems! I had her take out two mentions of 'kittens' from one poem. 'Cats' yes, 'kittens' no."

First Bogan lied. I did *not* change "kittens" to "cats" for this was a really *felt* poem about two of the wild kittens who both died, and the poem is not a poem for Hallmark, but really about our responsibility toward the animals we tame. Here it is:

> The two sick kittens, round-eyed, stare
> As if I were the one to be tamed
> Or give them what they ask by being there.
> Nothing between us can be simply claimed,
> But I, as nurse, can touch the heavy head
> With what should be a tongue but is a hand,
> And all night long they purr upon my bed,
> Their presence there at all like a command.
> Who can resist the sad animal gaze
> That takes us in so close always to fear,
> So close to pain, where violence obeys
> That deeper instinct that would have us near,
> And pays the price, for what? For human love?
> Whatever they implore that we must give.

But what is hard to take is the contemptuous "I *had* her take out" etc.

Bogan certainly gave me fruitful advice. But I was *not*, as everyone now seems to believe, her acolyte. She was never a muse for me. Because at the root of our friendship there was no real generosity on her part. Always the tone was patronizing, or condescending.

Later

I have now written the Greek family I helped for twenty years while their little girls grew up; Kyoko, my Japanese friend who was my guide when I was there in 1962; a Sister of Bon Secours who has started to pour out her life as she lies terribly ill; Marian Shields whom I also have never seen but to whom I have been writing for years. Marian sends me touching cards and messages and I admire her because she has kept her sense of humor, surrounded as she is by "dull people" in the nursing home.

Wednesday, December 31

THE LAST DAY of this bad old year full of illness, depression and death. I write that, it is the truth, yet it makes me laugh at the same time. For really, in spite of all my complaining, I am happy deep down inside me and that happiness turned into a short lyric two days ago.

But I am having to face at long last the unhealed wound of Bogan's attitude toward my work. She did not, could not, perhaps, respect it as it deserves. But does it deserve to be?

What all this does is to exacerbate and bring to the surface all my doubts about the value in the long run of what I have achieved.

Bogan was an extremely good critic but could not bring herself to praise me in print—as a poet. So either she was right and I have given my life to a crazy delusion, or she was wrong. And if she was wrong and perhaps knew she was being "mean-spirited"—one of her favorite words—then jealousy is the only explanation. Both of these possible explanations cause extreme psychic disturbance in me. At night I pace around inside my head like a caged animal who can find no rest.

It would help if the correspondence between us could at last be published. Bogan's letters to me are at the Berg Collection in New York and mine to her at Amherst College's library—in all about two hundred. But Ruth Limmer's hostility and sneering attitude toward that relationship has, so far, stood in the way. At least it is now understood in academic circles that she has chosen to do so.

Lately I have felt covered with wounds like a tattoo—everywhere I look in the past there is pain. Why then am I on the whole a cheerful person and as someone writes me these days "a life-giver"? Why haven't I given up long ago? What has kept me going? Partly I have to admit the need for money. I am used to giving a good deal—in this last week for example, seven hundred dollars suddenly needed when Medicare gave out for an eighty-six-year-old friend who has had major surgery. Medicare paid for two weeks in a nursing home. I paid for the third.

In these last years I have felt rich, but when I was ill I realized that I have been rich because I was producing so much. What if illness or fatigue, the fatigue of old age takes over? I have no large amount of capital. A year in a nursing home would leave me dependent. So the necessity to earn has always been a spur.

But deeper than that is that I feel happy when I am working on a poem. "My cup runneth over with joy." Sometimes the poem has come as the direct result of a wound. Everything is part of the whole person, so tattoo, an external pattern imposed from outside, is not an accurate image. The wounds, I suppose, teach—force to resolve, to surmount, to transcend. I will not be put down permanently like a dying animal. I can recover and go on creating.

New Year's Day 1987

AN OPEN BRILLIANT DAY to start the New Year, Pierrot, very affectionate, purring beside me at five in the morning—still dark—and the warm joy I feel when Karen Saum is in the house. She drove down from H.O.M.E. last night and we had lobsters—what an event these days—and the end of Maggie Vaughan's plum pudding—and sat with the tree and talked about our lives. Karen now has twelve students in her two-year college program connected with Unity College. Her eyes shine when she talks about three students, among the very poor, those to whom H.O.M.E. has been a lifeline. Imagine what being able to go to college means! A man who taught philosophy at Notre Dame but left because he got fed up with academic life is among the professors. Karen herself teaches history.

Off she went into the sunlight at eight this morning after helping me fill and put up the bird feeders.

Today the New Year feels heavy because I'm afraid my heart may be fibrillating again. I feel spent—not surprising considering all I have done through the season—but it is frightening, of course. It may be simply the result of a dry cough—I had laryngitis through a week of the festivities—and everyone teased me about my "sexy" voice.

I hope so much to be well in this New Year—to stay well, I mean. Last year was hard but I did learn a lot about Brother

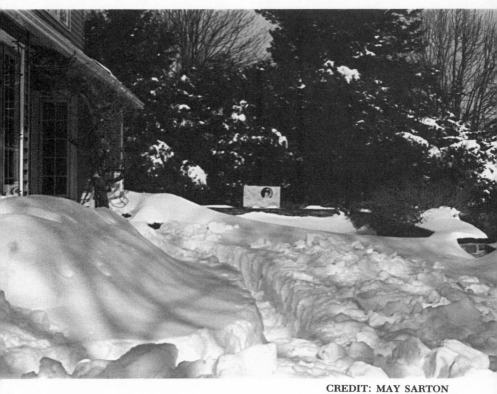

CREDIT: MAY SARTON

Ass, the poor old body and the heavy heart that somehow goes on beating, God knows why. Not a lost year but I am glad to turn the leaf now and look forward.

Friday, January 2

WE ARE HAVING a real blizzard, about four inches of fluffy snow now, but it sounds like rain and will make a frightful mess. There is always excitement and a fear in the pit of the stomach when there is a real blizzard. The fear is of the electricity going out. So I have put candles around and got out on the kitchen counter the wonderful small cooker which works on butane and also one Huldah gave me which burns wood alcohol and is less scary to handle.

There are to be tremendously high tides. Mary-Leigh and Beverly have boarded up the back of their house that faces the ocean she told me. They are terribly exposed right on the rocks, so there is also the danger of wind pressure on large areas of glass. I'm glad I'm up here on the Wild Knoll for which the house was named.

Pierrot is sitting on the table in the porch looking out at the birds and into the strange white world. It makes the house feel very dark inside somehow.

Meanwhile Maggie is driving her older sister down to Boston to meet a limousine which will take her to New York. Apparently there it is only rain. Maggie was to have come here on the way home and spend the night. I have oysters to scallop but they won't last another day so we'll have to see. Even in her Saab she'll never make it out here—and we won't be plowed of course until tomorrow when the storm has blown off to sea.

I'm going to have a try at the duck poem. Yesterday, too tired, I messed it up in trying to revise—too many words! Now to prune and test for accuracy. I want to celebrate these ducks which have been my delight all through this year. I see them as I cross the causeway on my way to town—often in a single line and very funny because they are so various yet so evidently "a family." The two geese are exotics with crests on their heads. The ducks are a pair of mallards and a white one.

Sunday, January 4

MAGGIE, INTREPID PERSON, did get through and walked in through the woods from the Firth's road north of the house, which had been plowed. It was grand of her to make it and a comfort. It is rather lonely here, I must admit, in a bad storm. I have only seen this much snow here once before, about fourteen inches and of course huge drifts. Then in 1978 it drifted against all the doors and I could not get out for twenty-four hours. This time light and power stayed on.

Yesterday morning, with piles of stuff to work at on my desk, I did not notice that Pierrot disappeared. Luckily Maggie was still here. For nearly two hours we called and she shoveled around bushes where he might have been hiding. I felt hysterical with fear—convinced that the furies were planning, on top of all the rest, to take Pierrot from me.

It was finally Maggie who shouted "I think I know where he is" from behind the house. There is a small cellar blocked

out from the main one under the porch where summer furniture is stored. But the door was stuck—open enough for
Pierrot to creep through, not big enough for a human being.
Maggie finally forced it open about a foot and a half and I was
able to squeeze through. A filthy dirt floor covered with pieces
of insulation the red squirrels had no doubt dragged in there,
some of which dangled from the low ceiling. I searched everywhere—no sign of the cat, no sound. Then Maggie came in
and was able to push from the wall a heavy wooden door, and
we saw Pierrot half-buried in the corner where he had tried
to burrow himself in, not lifting his head, in a state of stark
terror. I tore him out somehow and carried him in, filthy, his
fluffy tummy oozing with wet dirt, but safe. Would I have
ever found him without Maggie?

Last night I woke up around midnight and somehow lived
through his experience—felt the terror in myself—and saw
in a flash that he must have been chased there by an animal
too large to creep behind the door, too small to knock it over.
A raccoon? A coyote? A fisher? It happened in broad daylight.
But we had seen what looked like a large dog's paw marks in
the road when we went to get Maggie's car. Now I am very
relieved Pierrot has not asked to get out today.

I did do the duck poem but it is still not quite right.

Edythe comes soon to help me take the tree down, a yearly
ritual we each enjoy. I packed up Lee's crèche yesterday after
Maggie left.

Tuesday, January 6

YESTERDAY DR. PETROVICH's office was closed. I had hoped to have the nurse do a "strip" to see whether my heart is fibrillating as I fear it may be. No luck but I'll try again this morning.

I saw the sun rise, a perfect crimson globe in an orange sky in the center of my bedroom window. Only in winter does it rise precisely in the center.

Snow everywhere looks wonderful, so bountiful and clean. But how many animals I never see leave their footprints! From my windows up here I see swathes a foot deep, deer no doubt, and are the smaller tracks raccoon? Gray squirrels? The night must be full of coming and going but I never hear a sound. It is eerie. Pierrot is still afraid, stays out for a half hour and then is glad to come in and races up and down the stairs, in and out of the library, leaping up in the air in mock terror at a catnip mouse—flinging rugs here and there like a whirlwind. He is exhilarated by all the dangers outside, and having been a little frightened, then shows he is still Lord in this house!

I finally screwed up my courage to write Mary-Leigh a note about some small things that need to be fixed. The doorknob to the porch where I live and look at television came off in my hands two nights ago when I was calling Pierrot. He came, but I was nearly locked out because the front door was locked—nerve-wracking moment, but I did succeed in prying the door open. The back door's lock fastener falls out all the time but does work when pushed back in. The door to the other porch where the summer furniture is stored can't be locked since the huge rains we had before Christmas have swollen the wood. Little things, but they eat into peace of mind.

But then where is peace of mind these days? I am scattered into fragments of this or that every day.

Wednesday, January 7

YESTERDAY WAS A TUMULT of irritations but at two-thirty the rhythm strip at Dr. Petrovich's office showed no fibrillation. My heart is in sync still! I had been so sure it was back at its old tricks that I was bowled over. Wonderful relief.

I had felt restless all morning and decided to rush in to Jordan Marsh in Portsmouth and try to get a snowsuit for my godchild Heather Miriam in Knoxville. I had ordered one for her for Christmas and only knew the other day that it had been out of stock because my check was reimbursed. There was hardly a snowsuit to be seen, but I did find a size two, elegant, down-filled lavender coat reduced from fifty-five to thirty-five dollars. Staggering what infant clothing costs! On the way back I suddenly thought of taking some cooked shrimp to Keats and Marguerite. I got a pound which turned out to be a whole lot. Home at noon I read the mail which contained a request for a recommendation that Brad Daziel at Westbrook get his richly deserved full professorship and a request that I read poems on a cassette for the Carmelites who are being celebrated with a special Mass by their friends in Indianapolis.

I cooked and shelled about forty-five shrimp before my

lunch—and ate five or six for my lunch—awfully good! But these "things to do" weighed on me plus I felt terribly anxious about what the rhythm strip might show.

On the way to the doctor's office the car made strange rattling sounds. I thought it might be the shovel I keep in the back, but when I stopped for gas the old man at the station looked under the car and advised me to get help. Something was wrong with the muffler. It was then one forty-five, so I dashed out to Starkey Ford and they did have a muffler which they put in in forty-five minutes. Bill: one hundred fifty-four dollars. Money pours out of me like blood these days. But at least it is done and I can set out to have lunch with Keats and Marguerite today without anxiety.

I came home longing for rest, and did lie down for twenty minutes, then came up here and roughed out the letter for Brad's committee—also wrote a short note to Maggie Vaughan, including a page of this journal where she is praised which I hope will please her.

Pierrot follows me around these days when he only stays out for a half hour in the deep snow. Yesterday he was a treasure of affection but last night and this morning he is his old belligerent, macho self—he managed to knock my glasses off the bed table and broke the frame which Lee had glued together for me. I have a new pair coming from New York and am wearing my spare pair now.

I have packed the tiny coat for Heather and shall take it to the post office on my way.

What an interrupted solitude this can be!

Thursday, January 8

I SET OUT a little before ten to drive to Bedford to have lunch with Keats and Marguerite. I never got to them at Christmas because Keats suffered a long seige of flu. How precious it was to be with them again! This time they had prepared lunch. I brought shrimp all cooked and shelled for their lunch tomorrow. As usual we talked about the state of the world. They are deeply aware of all that goes on. "How shall we live with Reagan for another two years?" Marguerite agreed that Sam Nunn might be presidential material. Keats is reading the biography of Vanessa Bell.

I left bearing a bottle of Mouton-Cadet which they had kept for me since Christmas, beautifully wrapped in flowery paper. At ninety-four and ninety, Keats and Marguerite will not go on forever and this time I left them knowing how precious they are and have been for years—the elder statesmen one turns to for trust and faith.

I keep forgetting to say that at last I am reading for pleasure. Dorothy Jones sent me Patricia MacLachlan's small masterpiece—it won the Newbery award—*Sarah, Plain and Tall*, and I read it one morning when I was low in my mind, and found myself in tears. Such a pure style, such reality of imagining! And at last I am back to Jane Austen into which I dive every night with extreme pleasure. Keats does not like Jane Austen. "It is all about women wanting to find husbands," she said. This made me smile, it is so characteristic. She is passionately interested in anything about Bloomsbury.

When I got home at four the roof in the porch was leaking
again and the floor soaking wet. Luckily I bought plastic pails
last time. At the moment I am again in a chaos of the undone,
wondering whether my desk will ever be cleared again.

Later

A very hard day. Thinking of other people's needs—and
crying with frustration. I finally took five minutes to make a
few notes for a poem. Somewhere on my desk I found this
note: "I feel like an animal in a cage, and the cage is kindness.
The bars are what keep me in prison, what I feel I owe, what
someone else needs, the so much wanted *response.*"

So today the morning went up in smoke. It took Nancy
and me to manage to put a few poems on a cassette for the
Carmelites—for the Mass in their honor. They would *never*
have asked me. It took the best of the precious morning. I
wrote to a good poet in northern Maine, a woman who had
been badly beaten and forced to move away from where she
was living—sent a check. She is a good poet but unfortunately
depends on "pot" to write and so gets into trouble. I wrote a
Sister of Bon Secours who has poured herself out to me in
long letters and yesterday a cassette. I might as well say it
now. The letter by cassette *demands* three-quarters of an hour
of listening to a stranger. I can read a letter in a few minutes.
It is so imperious—this business of a cassette. I will not listen.
It sounds cruel, no doubt, but since my whole life goes into
responding day after day, where is three-quarters of an hour
more to come from?

It is certainly at present a life of quiet desperation. I am
nearly at the end of what I can ask of this self I bury alive
every day for the sake of strangers.

Friday, January 9

I WISH SOMETIMES I had never written all those books that attract people like deer to a salt lick. I am almost licked to death.

I couldn't sleep last night and around midnight I went to the window in my bedroom and was dazzled by the moonlight on the snow and the extremely brilliant stars. I saw the Pleiades rather near the horizon under Orion—it was thrilling. Pierrot often lies now on top of a suitcase which is held on the arms of a rather stiff armchair. From there he can look out and himself looks handsome, a white tiger. I wonder whether he sees the stars. He seems to be looking very intently at *something*.

Of course everything is brilliant in the snow dazzle since the storm. When I came home on Wednesday after Bedford, it was just after four and the sun was setting right in front of me as I swung onto the private road. It was a marvelous crimson globe going down and quite bearable to my eyes— an amazing sight through the dark pines and the snowdrifts.

Yesterday the cardinal was at the feeder again.

Saturday, January 10

IN BED THIS MORNING looking out on a very black sky, ominous, I read Alexander Brook's obituary for his mother Peggy Bacon. Rare the son who can so celebrate a mother, and rare the mother—and grandmother—whom Peggy Bacon was. She died at ninety-one.

> Her son, Alexander, in a more personal appreciation, remembers, "She was the ultimate creative person, recognized early in life, but rewarded only later with public acknowledgement of the merit of the great bulk and variety of her work and talents, never in the usual sense, with money or the things that money can buy. Neither ambition nor desire corrupted her. She wrote and drew and painted and etched and embroidered and the rest for the pleasure she gave herself in giving pleasure to her friends, only incidentally to pay her modest bills. To the world of her later life she was withdrawn; to the people she loved she was the ultimate giver, grateful for her friends, indifferent to critics, tender toward all sufferers, human and otherwise—an extraordinary person in her modesty, intellect, and sensitivity. Noble is not too strong a description."

After I came up here I was absorbed in planning what to say about journal keeping at Radcliffe on Tuesday. Suddenly I looked out and saw that the world had vanished behind a thick white veil—a predicted snowstorm was starting early! It was about eight-thirty. Because of going to Cambridge Mon-

day, I needed to get my wild old hair washed and curled—I
was in a panic and decided to fly out immediately and take a
chance that Donna, good friend and my hairdresser for the
past ten years, could fit me in somehow although my appointment was for eleven. It was slippery even then, with half an
inch of snow over ice.

Now it is ten forty-five. My hair looks fine. I have just
called Eleanor to read the obituary of Peggy Bacon whom she
knew well, for Eleanor owned a house with Cecile de Banke
in Cape Porpoise.

I remember how tiny Bacon's house was and how it was
packed with paintings, cartoons, embroidered pillows of hers—
a Beatrix Potter house it seemed to me. I felt she had a
wonderful sense of life, loving what she made, making it with
the total absorption of a happy child.

Wednesday, January 14

MY INSTINCT WAS RIGHT that the talk about keeping a journal
to a journal writing group in the Radcliffe Seminars would be
difficult. A two-hour session without material other than my
own seemed an ordeal. The backlash was severe. I do not
want to talk about myself except by reading poems. I am bored
by analyzing *why* I do something I do. I have never pretended
to be a critic nor an academic person. I had worked for at
least ten hours last week trying to put something invigorating
together and finding passages to quote. I hate rereading myself. But Dorothy Wallace who has always been like a great
warm sun—I used to call her "the sun"—had invited me and

arranged to pay my usual fee—and to put me up at the new posh Charles Hotel in Cambridge. How could I refuse?

I must describe the horrors of two nights in a glitzy hotel. I arrived at eleven—it had been arranged that I could check in early. A huge empty lounge. The woman at the registration desk did not say "Welcome" or anything remotely like that, but demanded that I give her my American Express card to copy in case not everything would be paid for. She did not say, "Enjoy your stay." In fact the atmosphere was frigid.

On the way up I told the nice luggage man that first impressions were all important in the hotel business as in any other. If people do not feel welcome they will not come back. I would not come back, I told him.

The suite was very cold, though well-designed. A round table with four straight chairs on one side of the living room, with a bar counter behind it, and a tiny bedroom with a double bed in it, and a television set and that's about all. I found it claustrophobic if I closed the shuttered door.

No flowers. During those two days I missed flowers and silence terribly—and Pierrot.

I had noticed men working in the hall and they made a lot of noise hammering and papering all morning.

At twelve the phone rang and it was Janine to say Marian Christy from the *Globe* was here and could they come up. Janine is P.R. for the Unitarian Universalist Association— which was launching a new magazine the *World* and honoring me at a reception on Tuesday and had set up the interviews. The front desk called to ask if I had an appointment with Janine. I realized why when she came up with Marian Christy from the *Globe*. Janine is black, a charming, sensitive young woman. I was furious. She had called me a few moments before herself to be sure it was all right to come up. The racism upset me.

I don't want to talk about the interview which was deliberately challenging, an adversary interview. Christy had not read anything of mine. Her questions were obtuse and domineering. A bad combination.

Finally at around one-thirty, exhausted and starving, I ordered a Martini, oysters and a glass of milk sent up—and prepared, after I had eaten, to lie down and sleep if possible.

At two-thirty a sharp knock on the door roused me from a doze and when I opened it a man was there "to put in a new sink." Mind-boggling. Was I so crazy that I had washed my hands without a sink? It turned out to be a round gold sink on the bar counter. It was soon done. A few minutes later I heard someone creeping around in my living room. I got up and found a bowl of fruit, cheese and crackers from the management. It would have been great to find them there earlier when I was starving.

At some point, I guess before the interview, I realized that the suite was icy cold. I called housekeeping and a half hour later a man came with a blanket and discovered the heat was turned off! By three it was very hot and I turned it off.

I must admit that once it was dark things warmed up— and the view was pleasing from the tenth floor, with a small piece of the river and a lovely sky to be seen between buildings. The hotel is built around a square, centered still now by a huge lighted Christmas tree.

Thursday, January 15

I FINALLY DID GET some rest and at five Janine brought
Rosemary Bray from *Ms* for an hour's interview. Bray is a
heart-warming, sensitive, highly intelligent black woman. The
atmosphere was supportive. She had read me, discovered
Journal of a Solitude last summer and went on from there.
We had an immediate bond as she was a scholarship student
at the Parker School in Chicago where Katherine Taylor taught
before she was called to be head of Shady Hill. From there
Bray went to Yale. Our rapport was instant and the interview
was a pleasure.

Poor Dorothy Wallace had a twenty-four hour virus and
could not have dinner with me, a real blow as I long to see
her. I had dinner sent up.

Tuesday was a killer and I am not going to say more than
that a five to seven reception in my honor at the Unitarian
Universalist Association on Beacon Street and dinner afterward nearly finished me.

But the saving grace was the drive from Cambridge to
Beacon Street with a charming Unitarian minister. There was
a full moon, the "wolf" moon, and all my nostalgia for Cambridge and Boston came back as we drove along the river,
looking out on all the lighted buildings, across the river, and
even criss-crossed the Hill to avoid the worst of the traffic. It
is magical still at night, especially since the old-fashioned gas
lamps—now electric of course—have been installed.

The brilliant scene was my reward and I was happy and

relieved to go to bed at last around nine. At ten I was half-asleep when a sharp knock came at my door, then another. I got up, rather scared, and was terrified when I heard a key in the lock and the door being opened. I shouted, "Go away." A man's voice said, "Sorry," and the door closed. I ran to the phone, pressed the emergency button and said, "Someone is trying to get into my room." "We'll send Security up," said the cool front desk woman. It took fifteen minutes. I could hear people conferring in the hall. Finally a knock. I opened to three men: a young blond in work clothes; the security guard, a black; and an assistant manager. They explained the front desk had sent the engineer up to check the suites. They had not bothered to find out I was in one of them! I was furious. It was then after ten and suddenly the exhaustion of the day and a bad fright brought on hysterical tears. I called the front desk and asked them to send a nurse or doctor who could give me a sedative. They did not apologize for what had happened!

Fifteen minutes later the manager and security came again to explain they would send for an ambulance. No doctor could be reached. It was becoming really hilarious, like a Lily Tomlin show. I said, "No, the last thing I need is an ambulance, but maybe you could bring me some hot milk and brandy." In a half hour they brought it and explained also how to double-lock the door. But I couldn't do that because if I had heart failure no one could get in!

Then I finally went to bed. A half hour later, another knock—the engineer. He thought the other two would be found with me! Incredible!

So that is life in a glitzy hotel. Lord, deliver us. I kept thinking of the Ritz and the Algonquin, shabby, comfortable, with beautiful antique furniture in every room.

I found a wonderful quote in *Newsweek* from Lily Tomlin's show, in a column by George Wills, curiously enough:

A bag lady is speaking: "I made some studies, and reality is the leading cause of stress among those in touch with it. I can take it in small doses, but as a lifestyle I found it too confining."

And now off to the vet with Pierrot to get his nails clipped.

Friday, January 16

HOW I ENJOY the daily drive to town! Every morning after three hours at my desk I set out, feeling like a truant from school. The road out is perilous these days because deep ruts of snow froze and have not melted even after a couple of days of thaw, but I look at the trees and the squirrels darting across the road, and the black shining of the brook that crosses under it at one point—where marsh marigolds grow in the spring. It is altogether a black-and-white landscape in the winter woods.

What I wait for eagerly is crossing the causeway and bridge into York, and looking for the flock of two exotic geese and three ducks who seem to be a family and are always together. Today they were swimming quite far off on the high tide. And the charming small buffleheads were diving nearby, such stout black and white fellows.

I complain about the mail and all it demands but it is always exciting to open the big box at the post office and see what is there. Today Doris Grumbach's *The Magician's Girl* which I shall start tonight, and a marvelous plush-covered hot water bottle from Maggie. I rested with it on my stomach— how comforting. The mail itself brought news that Sister Jean

has survived major surgery. I'm glad that I sent flowers yesterday. She says *Journal of a Solitude* has helped her through
the long wait. A dear letter from Blue Jenkins in Greenfield,
happy because they have a woman minister and Blue was
delighted by her first meeting with her. I felt quite lifted up.
Three or four brief notes of praise about my work. I steel
myself these days not to answer.

Today, because my desk is at last a little less of a chaos,
I can rejoice in the rich life I live, in all that comes to me,
instead of feeling like a camel on whom heavier and heavier
loads are placed as she plods through the desert.

Last night I heard three times the strange melodious hoot
of a mating owl. How can any female owl resist him?

Then, at six, early dawn, Venus was again brilliant in the
orange sky. Again I looked down on the snow-covered lawn
and saw how much life came and went across it that night.
When Tamas was alive he never barked. Was he unaware?
But the other evening the United Parcel man was gasping
when I opened the porch door, "A deer just rose up in front
of me," he explained, as though he had seen a ghost.

Sunday, January 18

IT IS SNOWING HARD and I feel sleepy and succeeded only in
clearing off a part of my desk—letters thrown away that have
been here for months. A little respite from pressure—in fact
a holiday.

Yesterday Nancy and I went to a movie for the first time
in six months, *Crimes of the Heart*, and as we always do, to

Luka's, the Greek restaurant in Portsmouth, for dinner afterwards.

Crimes of the Heart is the most beautifully photographed and directed movie I have seen in a long time. Extreme sensitivity to interior light, the light on the faces of the three famous actresses who play the sisters. I was a little disappointed in the text, written by the author of the play which was on Broadway last year. Nancy and I had the same chauvinistic reaction of being glad we are not Southern born and bred! Oh dear. The clamor of voices for one thing, like sharp bird voices, put me on edge. It made me long for Chekhov, for something subtler, less obviously dramatic—but in these days no doubt there would be no audience if it were Chekhov.

Wednesday, January 21

WHERE HAS TIME GONE? I feel I have been riding white water, Time a wild river over rocks. We have had another big storm, this one shedding four or five inches of fluffy light snow. So there are mountains of it piled up by the plow. It was two below zero at Nancy's this morning, she tells me, and must have been about that here. So Pierrot is not only an aesthetic pleasure, but very useful at my feet as a hot water bottle.

The cold and the excitement of these storms made me feel rather tired. Will the car start?

These last nights I have read Doris Grumbach's *The Magician's Girl*. A fascinating, puzzling novel which is ostensibly the story of three Barnard students in college and for years afterward, "the usual thing" one might think, but it seems to be really about monsters, why they fascinate. One of the women, Liz, is based on Arbus obviously. Minna is somewhat autobiographical, I gather, and through her New York City in the thirties is charmingly evoked. The third, Maud, whose strange self dominates the book, is a very ugly, very fat poet, a genius the reader gathers. Her passion appears to be words, not feelings or ideas, an interesting conception of the poet which did not really convince me—nor did her suicide. The last section of the book is Minna's teaching at the University of Iowa at sixty, falling in love with a young student called Lowell. Shades of Colette! I found this more convincing and more moving than anything else in the book. I think it is the most original of Grumbach's novels.

I presume that most novelists draw their characters up from the subconscious, not often as portraits of real people, though that does happen, but emerging from the subconscious where the seeds have been sown and then are fertilized and rise to the surface. Grumbach almost always uses famous, real people whom she has not known personally: MacDowell, the ladies of Llangollen, Marilyn Monroe and now Arbus. It is these mythical "real" famous people who fertilize her imagination. I find this strange. Feeding on an aura as it were.

Doris Grumbach is a very physical author. It is sexuality rather than sensuality which pervades her work and in this she differs from Colette. She handles it with great skill in the love affair between Minna and Lowell. The image of Minna at sixty as Lowell sees her as a peony fully open stays with me.

Brad Daziel comes for lunch to discuss his dream of putting together a "portable" Sarton. The preface will be his long essay (*Puckerbrush Review*, VII, 2) on my correspondents a really splendid job.

Friday, January 23

YESTERDAY A SOMBER, dark sky and the suspense before a big storm. As often happens, it was not as bad, here anyway, as expected, but the very high wind all night was nerve wracking. I expected the electric lights to go off and had candles and pails of water ready as when that happens everything stops: heat, light, pump for water, etc. Pierrot became wildly excited by the wind, once playing with a belt-end hung over a chair. He leaped into the air like a ballet dancer and did a pirouette. It was adorable.

A small incident at the hairdresser's has given me something to try to understand. I was there for a permanent. While Donna was securing my hair into curlers, an old lady who was waiting to be picked up came and stood beside us and talked cheerfully about herself and her daughters, and Donna responded. It was as though I did not exist, was an animal being groomed. And finally I said gently, "I'm a human being. I come here to rest." So the old lady said, "Oh!" and moved away. Donna apologized but in a tone of voice that told me she was angry. She went on working in dead silence. Then I suggested that maybe the way to handle it might be to introduce me to the other client. She apologized again. Then Chuck, the owner, said sharply, "Don't apologize, Donna, for what is not your fault."

So I felt like a criminal, a misbehaving child. I felt tears coming and bent my head far down, farther and farther, to hide myself away. I hunched my shoulders, trying to become as small as possible—feeling, I suppose, like a turtle, but I have no shell. Tears flowed down my cheeks. I wanted to run away but in the middle of a permanent that was not possible.

What is this vulnerability? It had nothing to do with who I am—but simply that as a human being one is hurt if treated as though one did not *exist*. And if this happens at the hairdresser where, of all places, except a psychiatrist's office, one should feel safe and sheltered, it becomes acutely painful.

I consider Donna a friend. I am very fond of her, a maternal young woman, tender with her many elderly customers. We did not talk about the incident but resumed our usual conversation after Chuck had left and we were alone. But I have thought quite a lot about it.

Sunday, January 25

ON THIS GLITTERING January day, glare ice on the road in, Susan Sherman is driving up from New York City to take me to lunch at the Whistling Oyster. I feel excited after these last days pent-up by the two storms, longing to "get out"—so it is a fine prospect.

I have had three letters lately that have helped me grow a slightly tougher skin. One from a Sister in Boston who enclosed an interview in the *Globe* which was inept and made me feel naked before the world, as no doubt I am. She says, quoting from the interview:

Regarding your comments about being "a good writer who happens to be a lesbian," I think that the goodness which is in our hearts and souls is what counts and not whether we are gay, straight, bisexual or God knows what. Furthermore, I could never imagine in my wildest imagination that God would label us!

The second is from a woman in upstate New York. She had discussed *As We Are Now* at a group. She says, "We have read about forty to forty-five books and I can't remember any besides yours that was totally enjoyed and appreciated." That was good to read but what interested me even more was what she told me of her own reaction to my books:

I wish to share two aspects of your life that speak to me and give me hope. The first is the acceptability (at least in some circles) of a female Muse for a woman. . . . I have been inspired by several women over the years . . . but never able to fully explore what those feelings meant due to their "unacceptability." Now thanks to your openness on the subject I can begin to look and to not be afraid of whatever feelings and Muses may arise in the future.

The second point I have found hopeful came to me as I was reading *At Seventy* this week. You said you are more yourself than ever. For that I rejoice, both for you and for me and all of us who need to be reminded that growth is possible through all of one's life. You have been able to grow because you remained open to others, and to yourself. When I am tempted to close myself up (which is often) I have you to inspire and remind me that there is little growth without pain.

The third letter—I've lost the address:

I could not, for some time, figure out why you and your work are considered "obscure." Finally it dawned on me that your interior freedom terrifies people. It is very hard to read your novels just for entertainment—put them down and say "nice story, now I'll get back to real life." You touch our real lives, understand the interior life too well for comfort, and force us to think. . . . You are courageous and therefore frightening.

Tuesday, January 27

SEA SMOKE TODAY, so it looks as though the turbulent silver ocean were boiling—because it is warmer than the zero air. Another charm of this brilliant dry cold weather is that when I sit up in the night to stroke Pierrot, down at the foot of the bed, his fur sparkles, rivulets of fire under my hand.

Yesterday there was a ton of mail so I never got to describe the delicious time Susan and I had at the Whistling Oyster. A bright cold day at Perkins Cove at its most glamorous with the bridge up. Susan remarked how like it is to a famous Van Gogh painting of a wooden bridge up like this one. Absorbed in talking and eating oysters, it took me some time to take in that ours was the only table with a bunch of tulips on it—and of course Susan had had them sent over from Foster's to greet us! She ordered a bottle of St. Émilion and as we talked and talked—really the first time we could talk in peace—we drank it all. But the splendid lunch was not all—at the very end I was presented with a small round chocolate cake, surrounded by strawberries to take home with me. Amazing kindness and thoughtfulness.

In the mail yesterday a letter from Juliette, such a delight to hear from her after quite a lapse. Her letters always bring me life, but what a hard winter it is in London! Her pipes had frozen one day.

I can't get the horror of Jesse Helms being ranking Republican on the Foreign Affairs Committee in the Senate out of my head. He surely does not represent the majority of Republicans, nor anyone except the extreme right. It is the ignorance that terrifies me.

There is a fascinating piece in this week's *Manchester Guardian Weekly* (January 25, 1987) by Marion Kumar called "Why Americans Are Different." She begins:

> Once again, Europe watches in stunned amazement as yet another American political web of intrigue unfolds. We can empathise with neither the actions nor motivations of the principals involved nor with the responses of the American people. We are learning, once more, that Americans are different; we really don't understand them at all.
>
> Ask a US citizen what makes an American what he is, and he will very probably talk about liberty, democracy, and "the American way." Probe a little more and it is likely to emerge that he firmly believes that *only* Americans have real democracy and are truly free. Moreover, he is suspicious of anything a little foreign and unfamiliar. To be "un-American" is not only second-rate; it is potentially evil.

That, of course, is how Jesse Helms behaves.

Thursday, January 29

A DELIGHTFUL PHOTO of the Carmelite Sisters and me when I was there in October came yesterday from Jean Alice, the prioress, and the day before a long letter from Sister Leslie, a generous letter as I had been rather critical of some essays she had sent me ages ago. It made me homesick for those radiant October days when I was the guest of the monastery, wrapped in a cocoon of tender loving care, like "a child of the house" as my mother always called my friends when they came to stay. I was homesick for the ordered silence, the pattern of the Carmelite "charism," as Leslie calls it.

And I was moved today to read her quote from Emily Dickinson, "We both believe and disbelieve a hundred times an hour which keeps Believing nimble."

I am now reading the biography of Krishnamurti which I ordered on an impulse because a review in the *Times* said that he did not *want* followers or any religious Ashram around him. Religious certitude too often creates a closed mind, foments a sense of superiority, *excludes* rather than includes, opens the path not to love but to hatred as is quite clear in the attitudes and behavior of the fundamentalists here in the U.S.A.

What moved me so deeply among the Carmelites was their open-mindedness, their total devotion to seeking the Truth even when it might be revolutionary in regard to Catholic dogma. They were never hortatory. They do not "have the

Word" against all others, they "live the Word" towards communion with all others.

There are numerous pine siskins at the feeders now, such a delight. Also the downy woodpecker and, alas, coveys of huge ravenous gray squirrels. But in the bitter cold, below zero at night, I haven't the heart to chase them off.

Sunday, February 1

I AM IMMERSED these evenings in a book as fresh and thirst-quenching as a glass of spring water, *A Maine Hamlet* by Lura Beam. It has been reprinted by a Maine publisher, Lance Tapley of Augusta, who is rescuing this remarkable writer from oblivion. Such lucid prose and such credible truth on every page. It is good that people understand that even today a Maine hamlet is not all Beans! In fact much of what it describes reminded me of North Parsonsfield and of Anne and Barbara.

On Friday, when another storm was expected with perhaps ten inches of snow, I dashed into Portsmouth to do errands and be well-stocked. The instinct to batten down and prepare for the worst is strong!

I bought the ingredients for a chicken stew, made for a change with white turnips, cabbage, onions and carrots. I got the car, which was covered in salt, washed and then stopped by the greenhouse. What bliss to walk into that green smell of things growing and to see rows and rows of primroses, a rainbow of colors, and cyclamen, a few azaleas, African violets galore and, surprise! two or three cinerarias. Of course I had

to have the blue and white one, one small brilliant red cyclamen, and two primroses, one blue, one a tiny bouquet, a
nest of brilliant red flowers with yellow centers. Oh yes, and
in my wild extravagance a tiny pot of purple crocus still in
bud. They have come out overnight.

The excitement of spring plants when the snow is deep
outside and wind chill minus thirty! But we only got about
three inches this time and valiant Diane came yesterday, managed to pry open the cellar door and take two weeks' rubbish
away.

The porch roof is leaking again, plop-plop, into a pail.
Nothing to be done till spring.

Monday, February 2

ROWAN TREE PRESS kindly sent me Robert Francis's *Trav-
elling in Amherst: A Poet's Journal*, for Christmas. I only
discovered it when I was tidying up the other day and read
it all through the night. Pure pleasure. I'm going to lend it
to Judy Burrowes who comes bringing sandwiches for lunch
tomorrow—if it does not snow! She is a good poet but like all
good poets gets a lot of rejections. So did Robert Francis.
Most people have no idea how hard it is to get poems published.

In 1931 Francis writes: "When a poem and I embrace, I
have a peculiar impulse to pray, 'Don't let me die, dear God,
till this is over.' The writing of poetry suddenly makes my life
of high value to me!"

The last entry, June 28, 1954: "Nothing can cure a poet's

malaise except to write new poems. He can't live emotionally in his past."

The worst thing for me during the months of illness was the absence of poetry—not to be able to write about Bramble after her death hurt.

Today again I am buried under the outside world piling in on me. A letter from a woman asks me to read her manuscript, a novel, and help get it published. One from a boy asking if I would sign one of my books for his mother if he sends it to me—at least he has the grace to *ask*! Two books of poems the authors hope I'll comment on for publicity purposes. Three gift books which must be thanked for. A long letter from a patronizing woman who assures me that the journals will live, not the novels or poems. A letter from the poet Roger Finch in Japan—which I must and want to answer. A mailgram from an old friend who has just heard of my stroke and begs me to call him.

A wonderful letter from Dorothy Bryant telling me, in answer to my letter about her great new novel *Madame Psyche*, that every character in it is pure invention, *plus* all the hard work she did about the history taking place in San Francisco from the fire, through labor wars among the fruit pickers, to what an insane asylum was like.

Not that letter which I treasure, but all the rest from unknowns silts me up till I feel crazy with frustration. What about *my* poems? What about *my* life?

Wednesday, February 4

WHAT A DIFFERENCE the afternoon light makes in February, a tender light I have not been aware of since September, a light that lingers on now till past five. A pastel pale blue sky with small lavender clouds floating along, over white snow turning blue as the light fades and the gradually darkening slate blue of the ocean. This afternoon I stopped hurling myself at all I should be doing and sat here at my desk for an hour reading Robert Francis's poems.

So I'll copy one here. It is hard to choose, as I remember when I was teaching at Harvard, a lowly instructor of English in 1950, how often I used Francis as an exemplar.

Invitation

You who have meant to come, come now
With strangeness on the morning snow
Before the early morning plow
Makes half the snowy strangeness go.
You who have meant to come, come now
When only *your* footprints will show,
Before one overburdened bough
Spills snow above on snow below.
You who were meant to come, come now.
If you were meant to come, you'll know.

Friday, February 6

THE IRONY IS that Robert Francis lived the life Robert Frost pretended to live and mythologized in his poems—for Francis was a solitary, lived on next to no money, grew his own food (he was a vegetarian) and had very little success. "What is more ludicrous than a successful poet," Louise Bogan used to say.

The difference is perhaps that where Francis lived close to the marrow, never married, and seems to have transcended conflict, Frost was always conflicted, treated his wife and children badly, must have known in his heart of hearts that he was terrible, a terrible person in many ways. The marvelous poems came out of constant struggle. Or the difference may be simply that Frost was a genius.

But I want to place here another poem of Francis's that does him justice. It is Part I of a poem called "Swimmer":

> Observe how he negotiates his way
> With trust and the least violence, making
> The stranger friend, the enemy ally.
> The depth that could destroy gently supports him.
> With water he defends himself from water.
> Danger he leans on, rests in. The drowning sea
> Is all he has between himself and drowning.

I decided to have a rhythm test yesterday as I was afraid my heart was out of sync. It only takes a few minutes and was well worth doing as the old heart is behaving in perfect sinus rhythm after all.

For some reason the cold got to me yesterday—that icy

wind that pierces one's bones even though the sun was out. Today I have on long johns and two sweaters. That should do the trick.

Jennings on ABC has been doing a segment on the homeless for the last three news reports. It does not seem believable that thousands of people five years ago or more were released from insane asylums with no provision for their future. The plan had been to set up halfway houses with some supervision. Without any follow-up, what did happen seems incredible. The federal government washed its hands of the problem and state governments simply let it happen and took no responsibility. We seem to be a Darwinian society now where the survival of the fittest means simply permitting the "unfit" to exist like animals, stray dogs or cats stealing from garbage cans. The dignity of some of these people is terribly moving as some of the photos last night showed.

Andrew Young, the mayor of Atlanta, spent twenty-four hours with a companion, disguised as a street person. What he felt at the end was absolute exhaustion; it showed in his face. One wonders why there are not more suicides.

The churches have done the impossible and feed hundreds every day, but they cannot do it all. They can't afford to build houses.

The key to all of this seems to be a kind of passivity on all our parts. We no longer believe that we can make things better. We have in an alarming way given up. I see it in myself. There is little in this journal about politics. What is the point, I have felt? And I have never felt as disassociated as I do now from the public realm.

Is it old age? Or partly at least that corruption in every area finally corrodes the human wish to be of help? Why bother? It is the age of crooks. The Democrats were wildly extravagant "do-gooders," we are told. Is it better to live as we do now under the aegis of liars and crooks?

Sunday, February 8

AT FIVE-THIRTY this morning the sun rose through a lemon-yellow sky, such a rare color of sunrise, and there were dark blue clouds low on the horizon—the morning star brilliant overhead.

One reason I am in such a fix lately about correspondence is because I know so many people, now dead, whose biographies are being written and the authors want me to write from memory. In the last week I have heard from Muriel Rukeyser's biographer, from Chick Austin's biographer at the Wadsworth Atheneum in Hartford, about whether I have more H.D. letters. Yesterday a query from the University of Science and Technology in Ghent asking whether I have copies of my father's dissertation!

The problem in all this is not only time but my own reluctance to look backward into the past when my mind is concerned with the present and feels held back by contemplation of the past. After the stroke I was flooded with memories—as they say a dying person is—and I found it on the whole painful. Much of the past is never resolved, for one thing, or one has resolved it by going on, by surviving, and in my case by writing poems.

I have not in earlier work said very much about Chick Austin's kindness in offering to Associated Actors Theatre, while I was director, the theater in the Wadsworth Atheneum. We spent a winter in Hartford and produced three plays. I had hoped to find a new American play, to discover a play-

wright but although I read hundreds of plays through an agent
in New York, nothing turned up. My actors felt cut off from
New York. We had too little to do, and the year was not a
great success for anybody. But Austin had been so generous
I regret that we did not prove more able to meet that chance
he gave us with a superior production.

Chick himself was a kind of magician as far as it is possible
to imagine from one's idea of a museum director. He had
immense style, for one thing. The air was brilliant around
him, but what is rare is when brilliance and style are matched
with imaginative kindness.

Monday, February 9

A BLIZZARD IS BREWING and I must run out with the mail
before it starts. Last night I had supper with Vicky and Glen
Simon and their family in their new house. They used to be
neighbors when they lived down the road in a big old ark,
and I have missed them and their two children, Saul and
Carie, now five and seven. I so rarely am part of family life
these days it was quite an adventure.

Vicky picked me up at five-thirty alone so we had fifteen
minutes to talk on the way, and just time for me to be shown
around the house before Glen arrived with the children. It is
a long house, rooms opening into each other, except for the
sleeping quarters, the children at one end, each with a room
of his own, and the parents at the other end, so there is privacy
in what is otherwise an open world. They heat mostly with a
single wood stove. The house faces south and is almost entirely

solar heated. I could not see in the dark the long stonewall
that borders a large field with the woods beyond.

Carie was anxious to show us the dance of the dwarfs she
had been rehearsing for a production of *Cinderella*. Saul went
off to make a journal—they have kept them in kindergarten.
Carie has written two stories. They wanted to show off all
these things and I was happy to be shown off to—up to a
point. Then I suggested that I love Vicky and we must have
a chance to talk.

Vicky had said in the car that her problem was never
having time to feel what she herself was experiencing. The
children preëmpt her almost entirely.

But as they ran in and out, we did have some talk. I had
not known that she had worked in a nursing home when they
first came to Boston from Minneapolis—but after two months
became ill from all the woe and bad treatment she witnessed.
But of course she must have been a lifesaver at the home.
She felt so badly about one old woman who had not been out
for thirty years that she and Glen hired an ambulance and
took her to the circus! Glen's firm is now adding a wing to a
nursing home in an old house in Portsmouth.

We had a beautiful dinner of artichoke soup, salmon, and
fresh asparagus, with splendiferous blueberry cheesecake for
dessert. How dear of Vicky to take such trouble.

The image I carried home with me was of Saul, climbing
into her lap as we talked and covering her face with passionate
kisses.

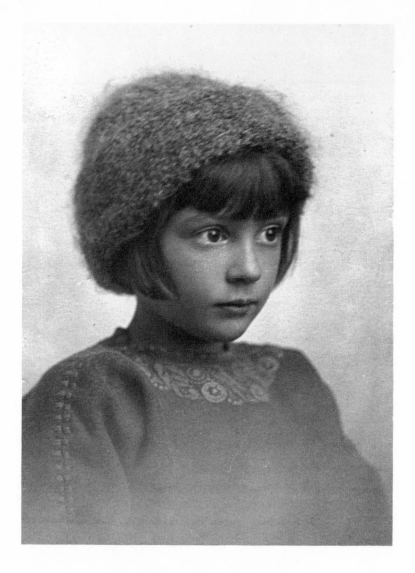

"A displaced person"—M.S. *at five*

Wednesday, February 11

ONE REASON I do not want to go back into the past, as when, after the stroke, I found myself in a maelstrom of memories, is because I am shocked that I could have loved so many people. Always when I realize this I remember Edith Kennedy saying once—not pejoratively—"You are facile emotionally." That may be true for all I know, but it does not feel true. I think it is more that I learned before I was one year old to make roots very fast, to attach myself to someone out of sheer self-defense. In that first year in Wondelgem in Belgium, I was taken from my mother at least twice and for a month also before I was two. My mother must have been ill. Once my father took me to stay with friends, the Tordeurs, and told me years later that I cried so desperately in the train, that he cried himself. It may be that my mother went away somewhere for a month when I was one-and-a-half, after the birth of a little boy, who died almost at once. That time her adoring, much younger artist friend, Meta Budry, came from Geneva to take care of me. She threw me up in the air and played with me in enchanting ways, and I fell in love with her, I suppose, for I cried when my mother came back. Such radical disruption before the age of two could have made me close up, but had the opposite effect. And when we left Wondelgem in August 1914, when I was two-years-old, our carriage riding through ripe fields of wheat, with gray files of Germans marching in the distance, the life of refugees was just as disruptive or more so. Because now for two years we had no home. There was nowhere to make roots at all.

And the beginning was traumatic. Belgian refugees were being "taken in" here and there in England, and my mother and I went by train to some "great house," where we were put in a cold isolated barnlike bedroom because I had a high fever, which turned out to be measles. The owners might have been kind but were not in residence and as it was, the servants treated us like unwelcome trouble. My mother got measles and was very ill indeed. And the only saving grace was the doctor who took me on his rounds in a carriage and called me "that topping little girl."

My father, meanwhile, was working as a censor in London. Mother and I escaped from prison—for that is what our quarters felt like—when farmer cousins took us in for a while and at last I had a playmate in Ruby who was nearly my age.

But at some point I was removed to stay with a childless couple. My only memory of that is being forced to take castor oil and my outrage about it, and the way it was forced down my throat.

What it all comes down to is that we three Sartons were displaced persons until we finally reached the United States in 1916.

And during the first four years of my life I learned to be charming, to attach myself like a limpet to a rock. My love affairs have been literally "attachments"—and when I have been happiest is when I could feel at home, and what I must have always longed for is family life.

The opposite of Gide who said, "Je hais les familles," I was in love with family life; it meant safety, a nest, a time to breathe and to be allowed to be myself.

When I remember where I have felt most at home during all the years, "Le Pignon Rouge" where the Limbosches lived outside Brussels comes first, and Céline like a second mother to me. She was fond of telling that she had held me in her arms before my mother did. There were animals, a goat, geese and ducks, a dog, a cat and a huge garden. There was Bobo, the governess, whom we all adored for under her German façade was a most loving heart. And there were four children, three girls and a boy with whom I could play. I was there with my mother twice for a full year, when I was seven and when I was fourteen. And I am glad I have been able to celebrate the life there in my second novel *The Bridge of Years*. After I was grown-up I spent a month there almost every year till World War II and many times after that. Now the house has been torn down and Céline and Raymond are dead, but I shall never forget any of it and her portrait hangs on the wall by my bed.

Friday, February 13

AT CÉLINE'S THE MAGIC was the garden and tea under the apple tree surrounded by Franz, the white gander, and his wives, the Persian cat, a few hens, and the leisurely talks one only has out-of-doors when tensions melt away in the evening light, when there is time to reflect, to listen to a thrush.

Grace Dudley's "Le Petit Bois" in the Vallée Coquette, Vouvray, was also home for me for several springs. There it was the silence, only broken by Jami, her wire-haired terrier, barking. Not family life but a wonderful quietness and freedom—the long mornings when I wrote poems upstairs and she disappeared perhaps to weed the old-fashioned roses she loved—the walks among the vineyards after tea—that order

and completeness of every day that is so rare. And for me—
and for her also—the passionate love we shared for France
itself, and the lazy, slow-moving river Loire—"ce fleuve de
sable et ce fleuve de gloire."

As soon as I lie down these landscapes from the past swim
up through my consciousness and I feel what a rich life it has
been.

On this Friday the thirteenth of February there was news
to set my hair on end. At long last the Ku Klux Klan is going
to have to pay seven million dollars to the mother of a boy
they lynched in 1981. Could this huge penalty break the Klan?
It has been reviving in Georgia lately after the march the Klan
tried to stop in Fairbanks.

I am reading proof of a new edition of Lura Beam's *He
Called Them By the Lightning*, and the story of her experiences teaching high school to black children in Wilmington,
North Carolina, under the auspices of the American Mission-
ary Association in 1908–19, struck me with great force. The
total racial separation is scary to read about. As a teacher she
had to be very careful. Negroes, as she calls them—"blacks"
came later—would not have condoned her becoming part of
the racist white community, and the white community did
not have anything to do with a "nigger-lover" as some called
a white teacher in a black school. It was an extremely lonely
life. It is a remarkable book.

It is nearly five and the snowy field is lit up to a soft rose
by the setting sun—the ocean very dark blue. The extraordinary beauty of the landscape in all seasons never fails to
"compose the mind."

Sunday, February 15

EVERY MORNING at sunrise three leaded crystal balls I have hung in my windows catch the rays and the whole room becomes a rainbow flight back and forth, over the ceiling, the walls and even my bed. Pierrot becomes a dancer as he tries to catch these light-birds, especially just above my bed. It is exquisitely beautiful and amusing, so I start the day laughing these days of bitter cold—zero this morning—and brilliant sunshine.

Tuesday, February 17

MAGGIE VAUGHAN came yesterday to celebrate Valentine's Day with me, a good catching-up time, but when we parted I had a wild fit of sneezing and one of those twenty-four hour violent colds set in. Yesterday I did something I very rarely do, gave up! Not a letter got written. All I accomplished was a final seed order and a lot of browsing in the Wayside Gardens catalog to try to decide on a small tree or shrub as a memorial for Tamas, where I shall bury his ashes. The problem is that there is a lack of space, the right space. I think I have decided on a mountain laurel which can be placed back of the daffodils and against pine trees—if it gets enough sun there.

What I did do yesterday was wander around the house, enjoying the valentine flowers, the plant window where Coleen's brilliant red cyclamen is surrounded by the azaleas I summer out in the garden and which start to flower in November when I bring them in. It is a dazzling show these days. Three white cyclamen have continued to flower also.

It felt very peaceful to lie around doing nothing—and today I am better and ready for my desk.

Wednesday, February 18

IT IS GOOD to wake up now at dawn, just after five, instead of burrowing down into my blanket because it is still dark, as I have been doing all during December and January—and the late light in the afternoon is dreamy. The dreams are of the garden. I have ordered as usual with wild extravagance about seventy annuals including all the old regulars: cosmos, nasturtiums, calendulas, Chinese forget-me-nots, love-in-a-mist, annual larkspur, bachelor's-buttons, shirley poppies. This year I intend to buy some flats, especially of zinnias and snapdragons because the season is so late.

The Wayside Gardens catalog is full of intoxicating ideas, but I try to restrain myself, remembering that ordering means planting in the spring and I must not pile up too much work. Sowing the annuals alone will take days. However, I am going to try their new Louisiana iris, and one or two roses. Except for New Dawn, which was here when I came and blooms all summer long and into autumn, I have not had much luck with roses. No doubt it is because I am so lazy about preparing the ground, digging deeply enough.

It is good news that Diane who gets the rubbish these icy days has agreed to give me four hours a week this spring.

How I look forward to gardening again!

Thursday, February 19

YESTERDAY JIM GILSENEN drove from Boston to have lunch with me. I haven't seen him for a year and he is thriving, earning his way through Leslie College as an English major— and hoping to do his senior thesis on my novels—and wants to teach as a career, and partly so he can teach Sarton! He looks like a Renaissance young man with long, very fine, red-gold hair and an incredibly innocent look about him. We had talked for two hours and I felt rather too tired when we came back here briefly so he could meet Pierrot who did finally emerge from the cellar—and came near enough to smell his shoes and look at him with wide blue eyes.

We walked in to a kind of apotheosis of things—a young man from Foster's had followed us from York bearing a single orchid and a case of champagne Susan Sherman had ordered to celebrate the coming to an end of this journal, the anniversary of my having all my teeth taken out two years ago and the stroke last year, *and* to celebrate my journey to H.O.M.E. the day after tomorrow to see a miniature wire-haired dachshund puppy who may be mine in May, and whom I have already named Grizzle.

There were also flowers from a family to thank me for my books—no address—and Nancy's report of a phone call from London from the *Times Literary Supplement*, asking if I would be interested in doing a review. Flattering, but I do not review, stopped years ago and do not intend to go back on that decision now.

Because I was tired, all of this made me feel rather bewildered and overcome.

Friday, February 20

VERY OFTEN in these last thirty years or more I go back to Freya Stark, a book of essays *Perseus in the Wind* (London, John Murray, 1948), when I am puzzling out something in my own life. Susan is generous in so many imaginative ways that I am at a loss often as to how to thank her. So this morning I turned to the essay on Giving and Receiving—unexpected and illuminating as Freya Stark always turns out to be:

. . . There is generosity in giving, but gentleness in receiving.

Of this art the Arabs know little. They take a gift and, with one swift appraising glance, put it aside, nor ever refer to it again; so that there is only a shade or so in general behaviour to tell whether they are pleased or no. The common emphasis on giving has indeed helped to destroy the receptive attitude in us all. Yet the one is but a personal luxury, a thing to be earned and worked for, an extra, a garland for one's own head at the feast of life: the other is a part of that general thankfulness which is worked into the very dough of which our bread is kneaded—it comes with every day of sunshine or night of stars: and gratitude is the greatest tribute which one human being can offer to another, since it is the same as must be offered with every breath of our happiness to God.

We feel this unconsciously, and love those people who give with humility, or who accept with ease.

Perhaps the accepting has to do with staying a child. I love presents, but not too many. But one of the things old age has brought me is being able to receive gladly and with joy, whereas, young, I only wanted to give, to be the one to send flowers and not to receive them. Susan is teaching me in her ineffable way to be a fervent receiver!

Saturday, February 21

A YEAR AGO at seven I was waiting for the ambulance with Nancy and Janice whom I had called at six. A long night of waiting as I had the stroke at one-thirty in the morning. I knew it was not a severe stroke as I could get up and I could talk. But my head felt very queer. I had managed to pack a suitcase, but somehow could not dress.

So this is the anniversary and I am well! It has been a long journey, but now I do not think about the past at all, only rejoice in the present—and dream of the future and a little dachshund puppy who will come here after my last poetry reading tour to California in April, and my seventy-fifth birthday on May third.

Then an open space opens before me—no more public appearances. There is much I still hope to do. And I rejoice in the life I have recaptured and in all that still lies ahead.

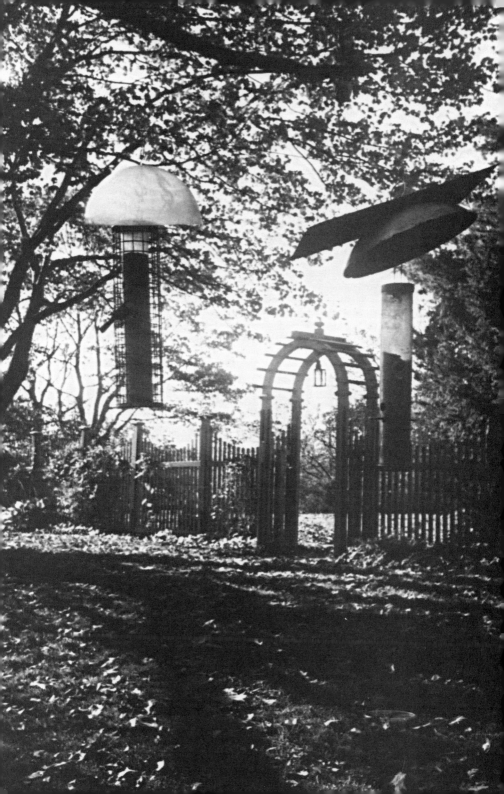